Mediterranean For Beginners

The Complete Mediterranean Diet Guide | Simple and Delicious Mediterranean Diet Recipes For Weight Loss

Table of Contents

Introduction 5

What is the Mediterranean Diet? 6

   The foods to eat 6

   The foods to avoid 7

The recipes 9

   Notes 9

   Breakfast recipes 9

      Summer Greek Yogurt Parfait with Toasted Nuts and Seasonal Berries 9

      Herbed Scrambled Eggs with Wholegrain Toast Avocado 11

      Fresh Mozzarella, Tomato and Basil Toast with Balsamic Drizzle 13

      Sautéed Tomato, Zucchini, Bell Pepper and Onions with Fresh Herbs and a Poached Egg 15

      Whole Oat Porridge (Oatmeal) with Seasonal Blueberries and Almonds 17

      Rustic Breakfast Baked Beans 19

      Frittata with Fresh Greens and Goat Cheese 21

      Med-Inspired Smoothie 23

      Salmon and Spinach Toast 24

      Asparagus and Potato Hash 25

      Feta and Olive Scrambled Eggs 26

      Med Breakfast/Brunch Sandwiches 27

   Poultry and Red Meat 29

      Meatballs in Fresh Tomato Sauce 29

      Pork Medallions with Roasted Fennel 31

      Stuffed Bell Peppers with Beef and Mushrooms 33

      Roasted Whole Chicken with Veggies 35

      Oven-Baked Chicken Thighs with Lemon and White Beans 37

      Chicken Cacciatore 38

Lamb and Veggie Skewers.. 40

Warm Beef and Lentil Salad.. 42

Lighter Lasagna 44

Pan-Fried Chicken Breast with Orange, Basil, and Almonds... 46

Ground Pork and Beef Chili with Tomato and Basil 48

Fish and Seafood 50

White Fish sautéed with Lemon, Capers and Herbs... 50

Baked Fish with Olives, Tomatoes, and Eggplant... 52

Grilled White Fish with Fresh Basil Pesto 53

Garlic and chili prawns with linguine.. 55

Simple Tuna Salad 57

White Fish with Chickpeas and Chorizo.. 59

Fresh Salmon with Lemon Butter and New Potatoes 61

Simple Grilled Octopus with Garlic Butter 62

Seafood Stew.. 64

Weekend Pasta with Anchovies, Lemon, and Chili.. 66

Crab Salad Cups 68

Mussels with Tomatoes and Garlic.. 70

Fresh Fish Puttanesca Salad with Couscous 71

Pan-Fried Scallops with Fresh Fennel Salad 73

Clams with Creamy Polenta 75

Legumes and Vegetables 77

Pearl Barley, Citrus, and Broccoli Salad 77

Creamy Rice Risotto with Mushrooms and Thyme 79

Herbed Polenta with Roasted Veggies... 81

Brown Rice, Feta, Fresh Pea, and Mint Salad.. 83

Whole Grain Pita Bread Stuffed with Olives, Tomatoes, and Chickpeas............................... 84

Beetroot and Goat Cheese Salad with Toasted Barley ... 86

Roasted Carrots with Walnuts and Cannellini Beans ... 88

Rustic White Bean Soup ... 89

Simple Weeknight Pasta with Olives, Tomatoes, and Ricotta ... 91

Quinoa Risotto ... 93

Artichokes Provencal ... 95

Eggplant and Potato Traybake with Yogurt Dressing ... 96

Bulgur and Roasted Bell Pepper Salad ... 97

Brown Lentil Salad with Grilled Halloumi ... 99

Israeli Couscous with Zucchini, Peas, and Feta ... 100

Fresh Watermelon and Goat Cheese Salad ... 102

Broccoli and Lentil Cakes with Avocado ... 103

Roasted Sweet Potatoes with Pomegranates and Red Onion ... 105

Honeyed Eggplant ... 106

Flatbreads with Roasted Cauliflower, Yogurt, and Asparagus ... 108

Mediterranean Spaghetti Squash ... 110

Cauliflower Rice Med-Style ... 112

Cauliflower Dough Pizza ... 113

Strawberry and Balsamic Salad ... 115

Tagliatelle with garlic mushrooms ... 116

Hearty Veggie, Bean and Barley Soup ... 118

Ratatouille ... 120

Roasted Bell Pepper Dip ... 122

Conclusion ... 123

Introduction

Hello and welcome!

What do you imagine when you think of Mediterranean countries such as Italy, Spain and Greece? I imagine azure oceans, warm beaches, relaxed days, balmy nights, and fresh, delicious food. Well, that's what the Mediterranean diet offers! A menu full of nutrient-dense, nourishing, satisfying and healthy foods which will improve your heart health, cognitive function and longevity.

I love that the Mediterranean diet is all about fresh, whole foods that truly nourish us, as opposed to restrictions and unyielding rules. When you take a look at the ins and outs of the Mediterranean diet, it makes a heck of a lot of sense. The "eat" foods are the kinds of foods you would expect from a health-giving diet, while the "don't eat" foods are foods which you intuitively know should be avoided. There are no nasty surprises or unrealistic rules, it's a "user-friendly" diet for lovers of great food, and I know you will thoroughly enjoy it!

What is the Mediterranean Diet?

The Mediterranean diet is based on the simple eating traditions of Greek and Italian cultures. It is a simple diet grounded in the values of local produce, simple ingredients, minimal or no processing, seasonal eating, and a macronutrient balance. It is considered a moderate-carb diet, with a focus on lots of healthy fat sources such as olive oil and fish. When you really think about it, the "Med diet" makes a heck of a lot of sense! Eating fresh, local foods which are as close to the source as possible, limiting red meat consumption, eating healthy, whole carbs such as bread and beans, and limiting processed sugar.

The mediterranean diet is great for the heart, as it includes healthy fats and Omega fatty acids from nuts, olive oil, and fish. What's more, the inclusion of fresh veggies and fiber-rich legumes helps to lower cholesterol and blood pressure. Fiber-rich foods are great for the digestive system and can help to prevent bowel cancer. Because we are avoiding processed carbs and sugars, our blood sugar is stable and at a healthy level, reducing our risk of diabetes and obesity. What's more, the nutrient-dense diet full of healthy fat provides us with abundant energy, healthy skin, and improved cognitive function.

The foods to eat

Vegetables

You can enjoy all vegetables! Aim for seasonal, local vegetables and create recipes based on what's readily available in the greengrocer

Dairy

You can enjoy dairy as long as it is full-fat, and preferably organic. Full-fat milk, Greek yogurt, ricotta, feta, parmesan

Meat/Poultry

The Mediterranean diet typically includes red meat or poultry once a week at the most. It is not a key player in the diet, and is enjoyed occasionally. Choose local, free-range, organic meat and poultry if you can!

Fish and Seafood

Fish and seafood is an important part of the Mediterranean diet, eaten in moderate amounts. You can choose any fish you can source fresh at your local fish supply. Preserved fish (such as anchovies and sardines) is also a great addition. In this recipe collection we also use mussels, crab, and octopus

Fats

Healthy fats in the form of olive oil, nuts, seeds, and tahini are included daily in the Mediterranean diet

Beans and legumes

Chickpeas, lentils, and beans are an important part of the Mediterranean diet, providing excellent fiber and energy. You can absolutely use canned and dried legumes! No need to start from scratch unless you want to

Grains and healthy carbs

The Mediterranean diet welcomes healthy carbohydrates in the form of whole grain bread, pasta, rice, couscous and quinoa

Spices and herbs

Fresh herbs and dried spices are an important part of the Med diet. Fresh parsley, cilantro/coriander, thyme, rosemary, oregano, mint, fresh chili, dried chili, paprika, cinnamon, cumin...any and all spices!

The foods to avoid

Processed foods

If a food item has been processed, packaged, and has a list of unfamiliar ingredients on the back? Put it back! The idea is to stick with foods that are close to the source, and close to their original state, without too many added factors. Avoid pre-made sauces, junk food, fast food, and supermarket snack foods.

Refined sugar and sugary treats

Sugary chocolate, candy, ice cream, cakes, cookies...it's all a no-go. These foods have been highly processed and contain lots of refined sugar that will spike your blood sugar, mess with your hormones, and cause all kinds of long-term issues such as diabetes and obesity when eaten without regulation. But hey, a little treat here and there isn't going to harm you, so don't freak out if you eat some birthday cake at a party or enjoy dessert on a special night out! Just make sure that your daily diet and your home is sugary treat-free.

Low-fat dairy

When eating dairy such as milk and yogurt, stick with full-fat dairy and avoid anything that states "fat free" or "low fat" on the label. Fat-free and low-fat dairy products have been put through processing, and often have a higher sugar content than full fat dairy.

Tip: when shopping at the supermarket, stick to the outside of the store. The outside of the store is where the fresh produce is kept, as it is easier to restock daily. Get your fresh produce from the fruit and veggie section as you walking, then choose your meats, then your dairy. Even better, buy your produce from a local greengrocer, your meat from an organic butcher, and your bread from the local baker. If your town or city has an Italian specialty store, you can find all kinds of goodies such as authentic dried pasta, anchovies, olive oil, olives, and cheeses that are imported from Mediterranean countries. A warning: be prepared to be overwhelmed and drain your wallet, as specialty food stores are like Disneyland to food lovers like us!

The recipes

Notes

A true Mediterranean-style diet will have the main meal at lunchtime, with a lighter meal at dinner time. However, the modern lifestyle doesn't always accommodate this, so do what you can! As long as you're following the key philosophies and eating the right foods, it doesn't matter how you balance your lunch and dinner meals.

However, these recipes can be mixed and matched however you please! You may want to take a recipe from the "Fish" or "Poultry and Red Meat" sections for your lunch. There are no rules at all. This book is not set out in terms of particular meals *except* for the "Breakfast" section. We all need a collection of quick, easy and nutritious go-to recipe ideas for our first meal of the day, so I made sure to include a dedicated breakfast section for you.

You won't find any dessert or baking recipes here, as it doesn't fit neatly within the mediterranean diet, especially if your goal is to lose weight. However, if you do find yourself craving a sweet treat, a little Greek yogurt with a few fresh berries and a drizzle of honey won't do you any harm!

Note that the Meat and Poultry section is modest in size, as red meat and chicken are only meant to be eaten occasionally, and in small portions. Some people require a little red meat in their diet for health reasons, so I've made sure to add some easy, healthy red meat recipes to keep your B12 levels topped up! The idea is to choose one poultry recipe and one red meat recipe to enjoy each week, with the rest of your meals filled out with vegetarian goodies such as beans, legumes, grains, and of course, an abundance of veggies.

Breakfast recipes

Summer Greek Yogurt Parfait with Toasted Nuts and Seasonal Berries

Start the day with something cold, creamy, crunchy, and filling. Remember to choose plain, unsweetened Greek yogurt. This is barely a recipe, I do admit! There's no cooking required, just some simple arranging. However, it's a great way to get into the swing of the Med diet with something incredibly simple.

Servings: 1

Time: 5 minutes

Ingredients

- ½ cup plain, unsweetened Greek yogurt (I used Cabot brand)
- 1 Tbsp chopped walnuts
- 1 Tbsp chopped almonds
- ½ tsp ground cinnamon
- ½ tsp honey
- ⅓ cup chopped fresh strawberries
- ⅓ cup fresh blueberries
- 1 Tbsp flaxseed oil

Method

1. Spoon the yoghurt into a cup, bowl, or dessert dish
2. Sprinkle the walnuts and almonds over top
3. Sprinkle cinnamon over the nuts, then over drizzle the honey
4. Finish with by piling the berries on top with a drizzle of flaxseed oil

Nutritional information

- **Calories:** 430
- **Fat:** 34.6 grams
- **Protein:** 11.8 grams
- **Total carbs:** 22.8 grams
- **Net carbs:** 19 grams

Herbed Scrambled Eggs with Wholegrain Toast Avocado

Any diet which allows eggs on toast is a diet I can get on board with! We use wholegrain bread, preferably sourdough, free range eggs, and a scoop of creamy, ripe avocado. This breakfast contains fat, protein, and healthy carbohydrates to provide energy, brain power, and satiety all morning. Fresh herbs completely revamp the flavor profile for bright, clean, multi-layered flavor.

Servings: 1

Time: 15 minutes

Ingredients

- 1 slice wholegrain bread, or sourdough
- 1 tsp butter
- 2 fresh, free range eggs
- 1 Tbsp each chopped fresh parsley, mint, and thyme (you can use any other herbs you have!)
- Salt and pepper
- ½ ripe avocado

Method

1. Get your sourdough into the toaster! If it's done before the eggs are done you can just press it down for a quick re-heat
2. Heat a non-stick pan over a medium heat, add the butter, and wait until it has melted (but not sizzling)
3. Crack the eggs into the hot pan and use a wooden spoon to break the yolks and combine the yolk and whites, constantly moving the eggs so they scramble as they heat (I am not fussy at all when it comes to scrambled eggs, as long as they're fluffy and not overcooked, I'm easy! If you have a go-to method, by all means, use it!)
4. Right before the eggs are cooked (*just* cooked) stir through the herbs, salt and pepper
5. Butter your toast and pile the herby eggs on top
6. Slice or scoop your avocado half and pop it next to the egg-topped toast
7. DONE!

Nutritional information

- ***Calories:*** 185
- ***Fat:*** 22 grams
- ***Protein:*** 29.8 grams
- ***Total carbs:*** 29.1 grams
- ***Net carbs:*** 23.1 grams

Fresh Mozzarella, Tomato and Basil Toast with Balsamic Drizzle

Fresh mozzarella, tomato, and basil is a combination too good not to enjoy first thing in the morning! We pile these heavenly ingredients onto wholegrain bread and finish it all off with a drizzle of tangy, sweet balsamic vinegar and olive oil.

Servings: 1

Time: approximately 10 minutes

Ingredients

- 1 slice of wholegrain bread
- ½ garlic clove
- 1 tsp olive oil
- 1 fresh, ripe tomato, sliced
- 6 fresh basil leaves
- 2 oz fresh mozzarella, sliced or roughly pulled apart

To serve:

- 1 tsp olive oil
- 2 tsp balsamic vinegar
- Salt and pepper

Method

1. Pop your bread into the toaster and toast until your preferred doneness (I like mine rich brown)
2. Take your garlic halve and rub it all over your cooked toast, and drizzle the first measure of olive oil over the top
3. Pile the tomato, basil, and mozzarella over the top (don't worry if it doesn't all fit, just let it tumble!)
4. Drizzle with olive oil, balsamic vinegar, and finish with a sprinkle of salt and pepper
5. Enjoy immediately

Nutritional information

- **Calories:** 335

- ***Fat:*** 20 grams
- ***Protein:*** 15 grams
- ***Total carbs:*** 25 grams
- ***Net carbs:*** 22 grams

Sautéed Tomato, Zucchini, Bell Pepper and Onions with Fresh Herbs and a Poached Egg

Time for a hot breakfast filled with fresh veggies and of course, a poached free-range egg. This is a great weekend morning breakfast, or for weekdays when you've got a little extra time on your hands.

Servings: 2

Time: approximately 20 minutes

Ingredients

- 1 Tbsp olive oil
- 1 garlic clove, crushed or finely chopped
- ½ red onion, sliced
- 2 large, fresh tomatoes, roughly chopped
- 1 large, fresh zucchini, sliced or chopped
- 2 bell peppers, chopped
- 1 Tbsp each freshly chopped basil, parsley, and thyme
- 2 eggs, poached your preferred way
- Salt and pepper

Method

1. Drizzle the olive oil into a large sauté pan over a medium heat
2. Get your egg poaching water on the boil now
3. Add the garlic and onion and stir as they soften together, making sure the garlic doesn't burn or become dark in color
4. Add the tomatoes, zucchini, and bell peppers and toss everything together
5. I like my veggies to be a little charred, but you may prefer yours to be more lightly cooked with a little "bite", so cook them for the duration you require to get your desired result (there's so exact science to this!)
6. Add the fresh herbs and toss them through just before serving, but leave a little behind for garnish!

7. Your water should be boiling now, so slip your eggs into the rolling water and wait for them to poach (I don't add vinegar to my water, I find it to be unnecessary, but you can poach your eggs according to your preferred method. Eggs are very personal!)
8. Dish the veggies onto two serving plates, top with a poached egg, leftover herbs, salt and pepper

Nutritional information

- **Calories:** 477
- **Fat:** 24.1 grams
- **Protein:** 19.6 grams
- **Total carbs:** 44.6 grams
- **Net carbs:** 32.6 grams

Whole Oat Porridge (Oatmeal) with Seasonal Blueberries and Almonds

One of the very best breakfasts you can eat (on any diet bar Keto) is oatmeal! Oats are full of fiber and anti-inflammatory properties. Plus, they provide slow-release energy which keeps you going all day. This recipe includes fresh blueberries and almonds. If blueberries aren't in season, use any fresh berry you can find! In a pinch, frozen berries are fine too.

Servings: 1

Time: approximately 15 minutes

Ingredients

- ¾ cup wholegrain rolled oats
- 1 cup water
- ½ cup fresh, full fat milk (you can use almond milk if you are following a more strict approach to dairy on the Med diet)
- Pinch of salt (crucial!)
- ½ teaspoon cinnamon
- ½ cup fresh blueberries
- 6 almonds, roughly chopped

Method

1. Place the oats, water, half of the milk, salt, and cinnamon into a saucepan over a medium heat
2. Keep stirring the porridge as it thickens and the oats become hydrated
3. Once the consistency is creamy, thick, and the water has soaked into the oats, the porridge is ready
4. Transfer the oats into a bowl and sprinkle the blueberries and almonds over the top, and add the remaining milk

Nutritional information

- ***Calories:*** 445
- ***Fat:*** 13.3 grams
- ***Protein:*** 16.4 grams
- ***Total carbs:*** 65.8 grams

- ***Net carbs:*** 55.6 grams

Rustic Breakfast Baked Beans

Beans are a fantastic way to start the day, as they provide excellent fiber, protein, and healthy carbs. This recipe is a cheat's version of baked beans, using canned beans (no shame in that!) and fresh tomatoes.

Servings: 4

Time: approximately 20 minutes

Ingredients

- 1 Tbsp olive oil
- 1 garlic clove, roughly chopped
- ½ onion, finely chopped
- 2 cups canned kidney beans (drained)
- 2 cups cannellini beans (drained)
- 4 fresh tomatoes, chopped
- 1 Tbsp fresh thyme, finely chopped
- 1 Tbsp balsamic vinegar
- Salt and pepper

Method

1. Add the olive oil to a saucepan or sauté pan and place over a medium heat
2. Add the garlic and onions, and stir as they soften
3. Add the beans, tomatoes, thyme, balsamic vinegar, salt and pepper and stir as everything mingles together and becomes thick and cohesive
4. Leave to simmer for about 10 minutes, or longer if you have time, adding a little water if it appears to be drying out
5. Serve!

Serving suggestions:

- A slice of wholegrain bread, a little grated parmesan, and a free-range egg for a power packed breakfast

Nutritional information

- ***Calories:*** 276
- ***Fat:*** 4.1 grams
- ***Protein:*** 15 grams
- ***Total carbs:*** 46.8 grams
- ***Net carbs:*** 33.5 grams

Frittata with Fresh Greens and Goat Cheese

This recipe is perfect for when you have leftover boiled new potatoes in the fridge. We cook them in a large sauté pan with fresh greens, eggs, and goat cheese for a special breakfast ideal for a leisurely weekend.

Servings: 4

Time: approximately 25 minutes

Ingredients

- 2 cups sliced new potatoes, cooked (if you don't have cooked leftovers, simply boil them in water until just soft)
- 2 Tbsp olive oil
- 2 garlic cloves, finely chopped
- 1 cup fresh spinach, finely chopped
- ½ cup fresh kale, finely chopped
- 6 eggs, lightly beaten with a fork
- Salt and pepper
- 3 oz soft goats cheese, crumbled

Method

1. Prepare your new potatoes, if need be
2. Drizzle the olive oil into a non-stick (if possible) sauté pan with deep sides, and place over a medium heat
3. Add the garlic, spinach, and kale and stir as they soften and wilt, add a little salt and pepper
4. Toss the sliced new potatoes with the veggies
5. Pour the eggs over the veggies and "nudge" everything with a spatula to make sure the eggs are evenly dispersed amongst the veggies
6. Sprinkle with salt, pepper and goat cheese and leave to cook until the eggs are just set
7. Either flip the entire thing upside down and slice, or slice it in the pan and serve

Nutritional information

- **Calories:** 292

- ***Fat:*** 18.5 grams
- ***Protein:*** 15 grams
- ***Total carbs:*** 15.2 grams
- ***Net carbs:*** 13.9 grams

Med-Inspired Smoothie

While smoothies may not be a traditional Mediterranean-style food...who says we can't get a little creative with the diet? Busy modern lifestyles require fast-yet-nutritious breakfast options, which include the humble smoothie. This recipe features healthy fats, dairy, and fresh green veggies.

Servings: 2

Time: approximately 5 minutes

Ingredients

- 1 avocado
- 2 Tbsp olive, avocado, or flaxseed oil
- 1 cup blueberries
- 1 Tbsp tahini paste
- 1 tsp honey (optional, but gives a sweeter taste)
- 1 cup fresh spinach
- 1 cup full-fat Greek yogurt
- 1 ½ cups water
- 1 cup of ice

Method

1. Add all ingredients to a blender and blend until super smooth, add more water if you prefer a thinner smoothie

Nutritional information

- **Calories:** 499
- **Fat:** 42 grams
- **Protein:** 9.7 grams
- **Total carbs:** 27 grams
- **Net carbs:** 17.8 grams

Salmon and Spinach Toast

This recipe is an excellent option for when you have leftover smoked or baked salmon. We layer whole grain toast with fresh spinach, salmon, parmesan, lemon, and olive oil.

Servings: 1

Time: approximately 5-10 minutes

Ingredients

- 1 thick slice of wholegrain bread
- ½ garlic clove
- 1 tsp olive oil
- Few leaves of fresh baby spinach (enough to cover the toast)
- 3 oz cooked or smoked salmon filet
- Small grating of parmesan cheese
- Salt and pepper

Method

1. Toast the bread to your desired doneness
2. Rub the toast with the garlic clove half and discard the clove
3. Drizzle the olive oil over the garlicky toast
4. Lay the spinach leaves over the toast and pile the salmon on top
5. Grate a little parmesan over the salmon (a tiny amount, about 1 teaspoon)
6. Sprinkle fresh pepper and salt over the top (go easy on the salt if your salmon is smoked)

Nutritional information

- **Calories:** 304
- **Fat:** 15.4 grams
- **Protein:** 21.7 grams
- **Total carbs:** 21.1 grams
- **Net carbs:** 18.3 grams

Asparagus and Potato Hash

Here we have another breakfast recipe which is great for leftover veggies, especially potatoes! Plus, it offers a healthy dose of energizing carbs and greens first thing in the morning.

Servings: 2

Time: approximately 15 minutes

Ingredients

- 2 Tbsp olive oil
- 1 garlic clove, finely chopped
- 2 cups cooked sliced new potatoes (if you have to start from scratch, simply simmer the potatoes in salted water until a fork pokes through easily)
- 8 asparagus spears, roughly chopped
- 1 zucchini, sliced
- 2 eggs
- 1 Tbsp finely chopped fresh parsley
- Salt and pepper

Method

1. Add the olive oil to a sauté pan over a medium-high heat
2. Add the garlic and cooked potatoes and toss as the potatoes become golden
3. Add the asparagus and zucchini, and stir to combine, with a sprinkle of salt and pepper
4. Slightly mash the potatoes and flatten the veggies down to form a loose frittata
5. Crack the eggs over the frittata and place a lid over the top, allow the eggs to gently cook until the whites are opaque
6. Serve with salt, pepper, and parsley

Nutritional information

- **Calories:** 340
- **Fat:** 18.3 grams
- **Protein:** 10.3 grams
- **Total carbs:** 32.3 grams
- **Net carbs:** 27.9 grams

Feta and Olive Scrambled Eggs

This is a Mediterranean take on the humble scrambled egg. We had fat, juicy olives, salty feta, and fresh tomatoes to free-range eggs for a protein-rich breakfast.

Servings: 1

Time: approximately 10 minutes

Ingredients

- 2 tsp olive oil or butter
- 2 eggs, lightly beaten with a fork
- 6 black olives, stone removed, roughly chopped
- 1 oz feta cheese, crumbled
- Salt and pepper
- Few leaves of fresh basil

Method

1. Drizzle the olive oil into a sauté pan or fry pan, preferably a non-stick one! Place the pan over a low-medium heat
2. Add the beaten eggs to the hot pan and use a wooden spoon or spatula to gently scramble the eggs by pushing the sides into the center
3. Quickly stir the olives and feta into the eggs right before serving, season with salt and pepper
4. Tear the fresh basil leaves and scatter over the top

Nutritional information

- ***Calories:*** 311
- ***Fat:*** 24.3 grams
- ***Protein:*** 18.6 grams
- ***Total carbs:*** 3.9 grams
- ***Net carbs:*** 3.9 grams

Med Breakfast/Brunch Sandwiches

These packed sandwiches are ideal for a filling breakfast or brunch. They're filled with tomatoes, spinach, feta, and eggs.

Servings: 2

Time: approximately 15 minutes

Ingredients

- 4 slices whole grain bread
- 1 Tbsp olive oil
- 2 eggs
- Handful of baby spinach leaves
- 1 tomato, sliced
- 2 oz feta cheese, stirred until it reaches a whipped texture
- Salt and pepper
- 6 fresh basil leaves

Method

1. Place a large non-stick frying pan over a medium heat
2. Add the eggs to the pan and cook until the whites become opaque and the yolks are runny, gently push them aside
3. Brush two slices of bread with olive oil and place onto the frying pan
4. Fry both sides of the bread until lightly golden
5. Place the eggs, spinach, tomato, and feta onto the bread (these are the bottom slices, so divide the filling evenly between them)
6. Sprinkle with salt and pepper, then lay the basil leaves on top
7. Place the other slices of bread on top to create two sandwiches
8. Use a fish slice or spatula to flip the sandwiches over (use your hand to keep them closed!) and fry the other side of the sandwich
9. The fillings should be hot, and the feta should be a little oozy
10. Serve hot

Nutritional information

- ***Calories:*** 499
- ***Fat:*** 23.5 grams
- ***Protein:*** 29.8 grams
- ***Total carbs:*** 43.9 grams
- ***Net carbs:*** 39.4 grams

Poultry and Red Meat

The Mediterranean diet is light on poultry and red meat. When meat is eaten, it's generally in small portions or as a side as opposed to being the "main event". The general rule is to have one red meat dish and one poultry dish a week.

Meatballs in Fresh Tomato Sauce

We're kicking things off with a classic dish absolutely anyone can make! Meatballs are easy, fast, and offer a modest dose of red meat. We serve them with a fresh tomato and basil sauce, and a side of pasta and greens.

Servings: 4

Time: approximately 40 minutes

Ingredients

Meatballs:

- 4 garlic cloves, crushed
- 1 onion, finely chopped
- 1 lb ground beef
- 1 tsp each dried oregano, thyme, and rosemary
- 1 egg
- ½ cup whole grain bread crumbs
- Salt and pepper

Sauce:

- 2 Tbsp olive oil
- 2 garlic cloves
- ½ onion, finely chopped
- ½ cup red wine
- 8 fresh tomatoes, chopped
- 2 Tbsp pure tomato paste
- ½ fresh red chili, finely chopped (optional)
- Salt and pepper
- ½ cup beef stock or water

To serve:

- ½ cup dried whole grain pasta (per serving), boiled in salty water until soft, but with a little "bite"
- 1 cup broccoli (per serving), steamed

Method:

1. Preheat the oven to 380 degrees F and line a baking tray with baking paper
2. In a large bowl combine all of the meatball ingredients with clean hands, or a very sturdy wooden spoon
3. Roll the meatball mixture into golf ball-sized balls and place them onto the lined tray, pop the tray into the oven and cook the meatballs for about 25 minutes, turning once, until golden all around
4. Drizzle the olive oil into a large sauté pan over a medium-high heat
5. Add the garlic and onions to the pan and allow them to soften, as you stir, for about 2 minutes
6. Add the wine to the pan and allow to reduce for a few minutes
7. Add the tomaotes, tomato paste, chili, salt, and pepper and stir to combine
8. Allow the sauce to simmer and become rich for about 5 minutes, adding a little water or beef stock if it appears to be drying out
9. Add the cooked meatballs to the sauté pan and drench them in sauce
10. Serve the meatballs on sauce on a small bed of whole grain pasta, with steamed broccoli on the side

Nutritional information

- **Calories:** 610
- **Fat:** 22.4 grams
- **Protein:** 38.1 grams
- **Total carbs:** 64.9 grams
- **Net carbs:** 54.2 grams

Pork Medallions with Roasted Fennel

My favorite way to enjoy pork is by pan-frying a lean pork medallion, with a side of roasted fennel. This is a simple dish which looks and tastes impressively fancy. Remember to stick to free-range, ethically-sourced pork.

Servings: 4

Time: approximately 30 minutes

Ingredients

- 4 pork medallions
- 2 Tbsp olive oil
- 1 sprig fresh thyme
- 1 sprig fresh rosemary
- Salt and pepper
- 1 lb fennel bulbs, cut into quarters, (lengthwise)
- 3 Tbsp olive oil
- Salt and pepper

Method

1. Preheat the oven to 450 degrees F and line a baking tray with baking paper
2. Lay the fennel bulb quarters onto the tray and rub with olive oil, salt and pepper. Slip the tray into the oven and roast the fennel for 30 minutes, turning once. We're aiming for soft, slightly caramelized, golden fennel quarters!
3. As the fennel is roasting: place a large skillet over a high medium-heat
4. Lay the pork medallions onto a large board and use a wooden spoon to gently "bash" them
5. Rub the pork on both sides with olive oil and sprinkle with salt and pepper
6. Lay the pork medallions onto the hot pan, nestle the thyme and rosemary between them, and sear on both sides for about 2 minutes or until each side is golden and the meat is cooked through but still juicy
7. Let the pork rest for a few minutes before serving with roasted fennel!

Nutritional information

- ***Calories:*** 439
- ***Fat:*** 20.2 grams
- ***Protein:*** 37.2 grams
- ***Total carbs:*** 8.3 grams
- ***Net carbs:*** 4.8 grams

Stuffed Bell Peppers with Beef and Mushrooms

Bell peppers are a fantastic vegetable for a multitude of purposes, cooked or raw. In this recipe, we stuff them with ground beef and mushrooms for a rich, filling, yet surprisingly light meal.

Servings: 4

Time: approximately 30 minutes

Ingredients

- 4 large red bell peppers, halved, seeds removed
- 1 Tbsp olive oil
- 2 garlic cloves, finely chopped
- 1 onion, finely chopped
- 1 lb ground beef
- 4 large Portobello mushrooms, finely chopped
- 1 tomato, finely chopped
- 1 tsp each dried thyme, oregano, and rosemary
- Salt and pepper
- Parmesan cheese (about 2 oz)

Method

1. Preheat the oven to 400 degrees Fahrenheit and line a baking tray with baking paper
2. Prep the bell peppers and lay them on the lined tray, set aside
3. Drizzle the olive oil into a large sauté pan over a medium-high heat
4. Add the garlic and onion and stir as they soften for a minute or two
5. Add the beef and mushrooms, stir to combine, and allow the beef to turn from pink to brown
6. Add the tomatoes, herbs, salt and pepper to the meat, stir, and leave to simmer for about 10 minutes. (Note: the beef and mushroom mixture will likely be quite wet, which is fine!)
7. Spoon the beef mixture into the awaiting bell pepper halves and grate a small scattering of parmesan cheese over each one
8. Bake for about 20 minutes or until the peppers are soft!

Nutritional information

- ***Calories:*** 363
- ***Fat:*** 16.3 grams
- ***Protein:*** 33.7 grams
- ***Total carbs:*** 19.6 grams
- ***Net carbs:*** 13.2 grams

Roasted Whole Chicken with Veggies

A roasted chicken is a classic, homestyle meal welcome on tables around the world. This recipe features a herbed butter rub, and vegetables that roast with the chicken, soaking up the delicious juices!

Servings: approximately 6

Time: approximately 1 hour and 20 minutes

Ingredients

- 1 large whole chicken
- 1 Tbsp olive oil
- 3 Tbsp butter, room temperature
- 1 sprig fresh rosemary
- Generous handful of fresh thyme
- Salt and pepper
- 1 lemon
- 2 large carrots, cut into chunks
- 2 large parsnips, cut into chunks
- 3 large potatoes, cut into fifths

Method

1. Preheat the oven to 400 degrees Fahrenheit and have a roasting pan waiting by
2. Place the chicken into the roasting pan and pat the skin dry with a paper towel
3. Stuff the cavity with a lemon
4. Rub the skin with olive oil
5. Finely chop the rosemary and thyme and combine with the butter, salt and pepper
6. Spread the herbed butter over the chicken
7. Pop the chicken into the preheated oven
8. After 30 minutes, take the roasting pan out of the oven and nestle the chopped veggies around the chicken

9. Slip the tray back into the oven and roast for a further 30 or 40 minutes, or until the chicken is cooked through and the veggies are tender (the chicken will be done if the juices run clear, and the flesh closest to the leg bones is cooked)
10. Serve with a seasonal side salad or some steamed broccoli and green beans

Nutritional information

- *Calories:* 671
- *Fat:* 42.1 grams
- *Protein:* 44.6 grams
- *Total carbs:* 28.9 grams
- *Net carbs:* 23.5 grams

Oven-Baked Chicken Thighs with Lemon and White Beans

This is a tray-style dish which requires only one tray. We bundle together chicken thighs, zesty lemon, and creamy white beans all in one! Full of protein, fiber, and healthy carbs.

Servings: 4

Time: approximately 35 minutes

Ingredients

- 6 free-range chicken thighs
- 2 Tbsp olive oil
- 1 lemon, cut into round slices
- 2 Tbsp fresh thyme, (leaves removed from stalk)
- 2 cups canned white beans, drained
- Salt and pepper

Method

1. Preheat the oven to 400 degrees Fahrenheit and line a baking tray or shallow roasting pan with baking paper
2. Place the chicken thighs into the pan and rub them with olive oil and season with salt and pepper
3. Lay the lemon slices on top of the chicken thighs and sprinkle the thyme leaves over top
4. Nestle the white beans around the chicken and lemon, and give everything an extra sprinkle of seasoning and olive oil
5. Pop the tray into the preheated oven and bake for about 30 minutes or until the chicken is cooked through

Nutritional information

- ***Calories:*** 495
- ***Fat:*** 30.2 grams
- ***Protein:*** 33.6 grams
- ***Total carbs:*** 21 grams
- ***Net carbs:*** 10 grams

Chicken Cacciatore

A classic Italian dish with chicken, tomatoes, bell peppers, wine, capers, and herbs. This is a rustic dish which means "hunter" in Italian!

Servings: 4

Time: approximately 1 hour

Ingredients

- 6 chicken thighs
- ½ cup plain flour
- 3 Tbsp olive oil
- 1 red bell pepper, sliced
- 1 onion, finely chopped
- 4 garlic cloves, finely chopped
- ¾ cup white wine
- 2 cups canned chopped tomatoes
- ⅔ cup chicken stock
- 4 Tbsp capers, drained
- Salt and pepper
- Fresh parsley, roughly chopped

Method

1. Place the chicken, flour, salt and pepper into a sealable bag and give it a good shake to coat the chicken in flour and seasoning
2. Add the olive oil to a large, deep-sided pan over a medium-high heat
3. Add the bell pepper, onion, and garlic to the pan and toss as it softens, about 2 minutes, nudge the veggies to the side of the pan to make room for the chicken
4. Ad the coated chicken to the pan and cook on both sides for about 2 minutes, or until each side is golden (don't worry about cooking the chicken all the way through, we'll do this later)
5. Add the wine and allow the alcohol to burn off for about 1 minute
6. Add the tomatoes, chicken stock, capers, extra salt and pepper, and stir to combine

7. Cover the pan and leave to simmer for about 20 minutes or until the juices are thick and the chicken is cooked all the way through

8. Serve with a scattering of fresh parsley!

Nutritional information

- *Calories:* 480
- *Fat:* 31.6 grams
- *Protein:* 29.3 grams
- *Total carbs:* 26.4 grams
- *Net carbs:* 24 grams

Lamb and Veggie Skewers

When you're in a rush, skewers are a total lifesaver. They can be filled with almost any vegetables you have, and little morsels of fresh meat. In this instance, we are using sweet, tender lamb!

Servings: 4

Time: approximately 30 minutes

Ingredients

- 1 lb lamb steaks, cubed
- 1 large red onion, cut into chunks
- 1 eggplant, cut into cubes
- 2 zucchini, cut into chunks (try to match the veggies and meat in size)
- 2 Tbsp olive oil
- Salt and pepper
- 1 sprig fresh rosemary
- 8 wooden skewers

Method

1. Preheat the oven to 450 degrees Fahrenheit and line a baking tray with baking paper
2. Roughly divide your chopped ingredients into 8 piles
3. Fill each skewer with lamb and veggies (don't worry if they're a little uneven, just aim for a roughly equal distribution!)
4. Take your olive oil and rub it all over each filled skewer, focusing mainly on the eggplant (they're like little sponges, and can become dry if they don't get enough lubrication!)
5. Sprinkle everything with salt and pepper
6. Take your rosemary sprig and bruise it between your hands, this will release the aromas. Press it over the lamb and veggies, this will give the skewers a little "kiss" of rosemary aroma without overpowering them. You can nestle the sprig under the skewers for further infusion if you like

7. Lay the filled skewers onto your prepared tray, slip into the oven, and bake for about 15 minutes, turn the skewers, then bake for another 10-15 minutes until the veggies are golden and tender, and the lamb is still slightly pink in the center

Nutritional information

- ***Calories:*** 376
- ***Fat:*** 23.9 grams
- ***Protein:*** 25.7 grams
- ***Total carbs:*** 16.6 grams
- ***Net carbs:*** 10.2 grams

Warm Beef and Lentil Salad

This salad can be tossed together quickly and with minimal effort aside from grilling a piece of juicy steak. We toss sliced, warm beef with lentils, feta, mint, lemon, and parsley. It's a refreshing, Summery salad which can be eaten with one bowl, one fork, and preferably a wee glass of red wine!

Servings: 4

Time: approximately 25 minutes

Ingredients

- 1 large piece of steak, (rump steak is great), about 1 lb, room temperature
- 1 Tbsp olive oil
- Salt and pepper
- 3 cups canned brown lentils, (3 cups once drained)
- ½ red onion, finely chopped
- 3 oz feta cheese, crumbled
- ½ cup finely chopped parsley
- ⅓ cup finely chopped mint
- Juice of 1 lemon
- 3 Tbsp olive oil

Method

1. Place a skillet over a high heat
2. Rub the steak with olive oil and sprinkle with salt and pepper
3. Lay the steak onto the hot skillet and sear on both sides until golden, but still blushing in the center (medium rare), leave to rest while you prepare the salad
4. In a large salad bowl, toss the lentils, onion, feta, parsley, mint, lemon juice, and olive oil
5. Slice the warm steak into thin slices and lay on top of the salad, or divide individually when serving

Nutritional information

- ***Calories:*** 442
- ***Fat:*** 21.3 grams

- ***Protein:*** 39.3 grams
- ***Total carbs:*** 24.8 grams
- ***Net carbs:*** 18.4 grams

Lighter Lasagna

Who doesn't love lasagna!? This lasagna is a lighter version, so you can enjoy the classic flavor and comforting aroma without feeling heavy or weighed down afterward.

Servings: 6

Time: approximately 1 hour

Ingredients

- 2 Tbsp olive oil
- 1 onion, finely chopped
- 4 garlic cloves, finely chopped
- 1 ½ lbs ground beef
- ⅓ cup red wine
- 2 cups canned chopped tomatoes
- 1 tsp dried chili flakes
- 1 tsp each dried oregano, thyme, and rosemary
- Salt and pepper
- 12 sheets (12 halves or 6 whole sheets) fresh lasagna (enough to create three layers across the entire dish)
- Large handful of fresh basil
- 5 oz fresh mozzarella, torn

Method

1. Add the olive oil to a large sauté pan over a medium-high heat
2. Add the onion and garlic to the pan and stir as they soften for about 2 minutes
3. Add the beef and stir as it turns from pink to brown
4. Add the red wine and allow the alcohol to burn off for about 2 minutes
5. Add the tomatoes, chili flakes, herbs, salt and pepper and stir to combine
6. Leave to simmer for about 30 minutes until thick and rich in flavor
7. Preheat the oven to 400 degrees Fahrenheit and have a lasagna dish waiting by
8. Layer the lasagna in this fashion: start with a layer of beef mixture on the bottom, then a layer of pasta, then a few torn basil leaves, repeat until everything has been used, and the top layer

is beef sauce (it's not meant to be super tidy, just throw it all together as you please, as long as it's roughly even!)

9. Finish with the torn mozzarella and a few extra basil leaves
10. Bake in the oven for about 30 minutes or until everything is golden and bubbling

Nutritional information

- *Calories:* 714
- *Fat:* 34 grams
- *Protein:* 50.5 grams
- *Total carbs:* 47.1 grams
- *Net carbs:* 41 grams

Pan-Fried Chicken Breast with Orange, Basil, and Almonds

This recipe is a great way to get the benefits of chicken breast (lean protein!) in a simple and quick way. We use fresh orange juice and basil leaves for a sweet and aromatic flavor profile. Chopped almonds provide crunch, nuttiness, and healthy fats

Servings: 4

Time: approximately 30 minutes

Ingredients

- 2 Tbsp olive oil
- 1 Tbsp butter
- 2 garlic cloves, finely chopped
- 1 red onion, finely chopped
- 2 large chicken breasts, skin removed
- Juice of 1 orange
- Large handful of fresh basil, roughly chopped
- ½ cup chopped raw almonds
- Salt and pepper

Method

1. Place the chicken breasts between two sheets of baking paper and use a rolling pin to bash them down so that they are even in thickness (about ½ cm)
2. Add the olive oil and butter to a large sauté pan over a medium-high heat
3. Add the garlic and onion to the pan and stir as they soften
4. Add the chicken breasts to the pan and sear on both sides until golden and almost cooked through
5. Add the ~~lemon~~ *orange* juice, basil, almonds, salt, and pepper to the pan and use a wooden spoon to remove the "sticky bits" from the bottom of the pan (these are full of flavor!), and cook the chicken ~~right~~ *all* the way through
6. Serve with a side salad, steamed greens, or even a side of pasta

Nutritional information

- **Calories:** 334

- *Fat:* 19.6 grams
- *Protein:* 39.3 grams
- *Total carbs:* 9.6 grams
- *Net carbs:* 6.8 grams

Ground Pork and Beef Chili with Tomato and Basil

Ground meat is a lifesaver when it comes to making fast, easy, and nutritious meals. This recipe is a Mediterranean version of a classic chili, with tomatoes, basil, and a sprinkling of parmesan cheese. It's part Bolognese, part chili!

Servings: 5

Time: approximately 30 minutes

Ingredients

- 3 Tbsp olive oil
- 1 large onion, finely chopped
- 5 garlic cloves, finely chopped
- 1 tsp dried red chili flakes
- 2 red bell peppers, finely chopped
- 1 lb ground beef
- 1 lb ground pork
- ½ cup red wine
- 3 cups canned chopped tomatoes
- ½ cup roughly chopped fresh basil
- Salt and pepper

Method

1. Add the olive oil to a large sauté pan over a medium-high heat
2. Add the onions, garlic, chili, and bell peppers and stir as they soften together, for about 3 minutes
3. Add the pork and beef and stir as they turn from pink to brown
4. Add the wine and allow the alcohol to burn off for about 2 minutes
5. Add the tomatoes, basil, salt and pepper, cover and allow to simmer for about 15 minutes. If it appears to be drying out, add a little water!
6. Serve hot, with brown rice pasta, or a side salad

Nutritional information

- **Calories:** 589

- *Fat:* 36.9 grams
- *Protein:* 44.5 grams
- *Total carbs:* 14.4 grams
- *Net carbs:* 12.5 grams

Fish and Seafood

Fish and seafood is a major part of the Mediterranean diet (makes sense, considering all of that luscious ocean on the doorstep!). Fish and seafood provides excellent protein and healthy fats. These recipes include salmon, tuna, white fish, mussels, prawns, and crab. When it comes to white fish filets, use whatever variety of fresh fish you can source in your region.

White Fish sautéed with Lemon, Capers and Herbs

One of the best ways to prepare a filet of fresh white fish is to simply pan-fry it with lemon, capers, and fresh herbs. The combination of sourness, aromatic freshness, and briny saltiness brings so much life to the fish!

Servings: 4

Time: approximately 20 minutes

Ingredients

- 2 Tbsp olive oil
- 2 Tbsp butter
- 4 large fresh fish fillets
- Juice of 2 large lemons
- 3 Tbsp capers
- ½ cup chopped fresh parsley, mint, thyme (or any other fresh herbs you like)
- Salt and pepper

Method

1. Place a non-stick pan over a medium-high heat and add the olive oil and butter, allow the butter to melt and become slightly frothy
2. Add the fish to the pan and fry on both sides for about 2 minutes or until golden and almost cooked through
3. Add the lemon juice and capers, and allow the acid of the lemon juice to deglaze the pan
4. Add the fresh herbs just before you remove the pan from the heat and serve
5. Serve with a little extra butter and a wedge of lemon!

Nutritional information

- ***Calories:*** 282
- ***Fat:*** 15 grams
- ***Protein:*** 35.2 grams
- ***Total carbs:*** 2.9 grams
- ***Net carbs:*** 2.6 grams

Baked Fish with Olives, Tomatoes, and Eggplant

This is an easy dish requiring only one dish, in which we bake fresh white fish, briny olives, rich tomatoes, and soft eggplant.

Servings: 4

Time: approximately 35 minutes

Ingredients

- 1 eggplant, thinly sliced
- 4 Tbsp olive oil
- Salt and pepper
- 4 large, fresh white fish fillets
- 2 cups canned whole tomatoes
- 20 black olives, (remove the stones if you wish, but not crucial)
- Fresh parsley

Method

1. Preheat the oven to 360 degrees Fahrenheit
2. Lay the eggplant into the bottom of a baking dish, and drizzle each slice with olive oil, salt and pepper and make sure each slice is coated
3. Pour half of the tomatoes over the eggplant
4. Lay the fish onto the tomatoes and add the other half of the tomatoes over the top
5. Scatter the olives over the tomatoes and pop the dish into the oven to bake for about 30 minutes or until the eggplant is soft and the fish is just cooked through
6. Serve hot, with a scattering of fresh parsley

Nutritional information

- ***Calories:*** 481
- ***Fat:*** 19 grams
- ***Protein:*** 60.3 grams
- ***Total carbs:*** 15.1 grams
- ***Net carbs:*** 9 grams

Grilled White Fish with Fresh Basil Pesto

This is an easy dish to whip up when you want to impress guests without putting in too much effort. Fresh, homemade pesto is surprisingly easy to make! You just need a decent bunch of fresh, fragrant basil.

Servings: 4

Time: approximately 30 minutes

Ingredients

Pesto:

- 1 cup fresh basil leaves
- 4 Tbsp olive oil
- ¼ cup grated parmesan
- ¼ cup toasted pine nuts
- Juice of ½ lemon
- Salt and pepper
- 4 fresh white fish fillets

Method

1. Place the pesto ingredients into a food processor and blitz until smooth
2. Place the pesto into a bowl, and add the fish filets, ensuring each one is coated in pesto
3. Place a griddle pan onto a high heat
4. Place the pesto-coated fish filets onto the hot griddle pan and grill on both sides until slightly charred, and the fish is cooked through but still juicy
5. Serve the fish with the leftover pesto on top

Serving suggestion: a side of steamed new potatoes with butter, salt and pepper

Nutritional information

- **Calories:** 488
- **Fat:** 24.9 grams
- **Protein:** 61.9 grams
- **Total carbs:** 1.6 grams

- ***Net carbs:*** 1.1 grams

Garlic and chili prawns with linguine

This dish is a real crowd-pleaser, especially for seafood lovers. We cook prawns over high heat with garlic and chili, and toss them with fresh, al dente linguine.

Servings: 4

Time: approximately 35 minutes

Ingredients

- 2 Tbsp olive oil
- 1 Tbsp butter
- 4 garlic cloves, finely chopped
- 1 fresh red chili, finely chopped
- 1 lb prawns, cleaned
- 1 ½ lbs dry linguine
- ½ cup grated parmesan cheese
- Zest of 1 lemon
- Large handful fresh parsley, roughly chopped

Method

1. Fill a pasta pot with very salty water, cover, and allow to boil, add the linguine
2. Place a large sauté pan over a high heat and add the olive oil and butter
3. Add the prawns, garlic, and chili and toss as the prawns cook through, turn down the heat
4. Transfer the cooked linguine to the pan with the prawns, transferring some of the pasta water as you do so, use tongs to toss everything together
5. Add the lemon juice, parmesan, and parsley right before serving and quickly toss to combine
6. Serve hot!

Nutritional information

- ***Calories:*** 851
- ***Fat:*** 15.9 grams
- ***Protein:*** 49.2 grams
- ***Total carbs:*** 129.4 grams

- ***Net carbs:*** 120 grams

Simple Tuna Salad

This is a delicious salad filled with fresh, crispy veggies and protein-rich tuna and eggs. We cheat a little by using canned tuna, but there's no shame in that! The only cooking involved is boiling a couple of eggs.

Servings: 4

Time: approximately 20 minutes

Ingredients

- 8 cups crispy cos lettuce, roughly shredded
- 2 large tomatoes, cut into chunks
- 2 cup cucumber cubes
- 2 carrots, cut into small pieces
- 1 cup sliced radishes
- 1 avocado, cut into chunks
- 4 eggs
- 14 oz canned tuna, in olive oil, drained
- Juice of 1 lemon
- 1 tsp mustard
- 3 Tbsp olive oil
- Salt and pepper

Method

1. Bring a pot of water (just enough to cover an egg) to a rolling boil
2. Use a slotted spoon to lower the four eggs into the water and set the timer for 10 minutes
3. Gently drain the hot water out of the saucepan and refill it with cold water to allow the eggs to cool down for about 5 minutes
4. Assemble the lettuce, tomatoes, cucumber, carrots, radishes, and avocado into four serving bowls
5. Peel the eggs and cut each one into quarters, and divide between the four bowls
6. Flake the tuna onto the salads
7. In a small cup or bowl, mix together the lemon, mustard, olive oil, salt and pepper

8. Drizzle the dressing over the salads right before serving

Nutritional information

- ***Calories:*** 499
- ***Fat:*** 34.9 grams
- ***Protein:*** 31.5 grams
- ***Total carbs:*** 17 grams
- ***Net carbs:*** 10.2 grams

White Fish with Chickpeas and Chorizo

The smoky flavor of chorizo infuses white fish, with the creamy, filling addition of chickpeas.

Servings: 4

Time: approximately 30 minutes

Ingredients

- 2 Tbsp olive oil
- 4 garlic cloves, finely chopped
- 1 onion, finely chopped
- 2 tsp paprika
- ½ tsp chili powder
- 5 oz chorizo sausage, sliced
- 4 large white fresh fish filets
- 2 cups canned chickpeas (2 cups once drained)
- 3 large fresh tomatoes, cut into small pieces
- Salt and pepper
- Fresh coriander/cilantro

Method

1. Place a large sauté pan over a medium-high heat and add the olive oil
2. Add the garlic and onions to the pan and stir as they soften and become fragrant
3. Add the paprika, chili, and paprika and stir as the fat in the paprika melts away and the pieces become golden
4. Shuffle the ingredients in the pan aside to make room for the fish
5. Add the fish filets to the pan and sprinkle each side with salt and pepper
6. Cook the fish for about 2 minutes each side until golden
7. Add the tomatoes and chickpeas to the pan, add more salt and pepper, cover the pan and leave to cook for about 5 minutes
8. Serve hot, with a generous scattering of coriander/cilantro!

Nutritional information

- ***Calories:*** 460
- ***Fat:*** 18.9 grams
- ***Protein:*** 50.6 grams
- ***Total carbs:*** 28.5 grams
- ***Net carbs:*** 19.7 grams

Fresh Salmon with Lemon Butter and New Potatoes

What's better than a dinner of fresh salmon, cooked with lemony butter and served with steaming, hot new potatoes? Summer in a dish.

Servings: 4

Time: approximately 30 minutes

Ingredients

- 4 filets fresh salmon
- 2 lemons, thinly sliced
- 2 Tbsp butter
- Salt and pepper
- Fresh parsley, finely chopped
- 1 ½ lbs new potatoes, halved if they are large, just aim for even-sized pieces

Method

1. Preheat the oven to 400 degrees Fahrenheit and line a baking tray with baking paper
2. Place the salmon onto the tray and rub each fillet with butter, and sprinkle each with salt and pepper
3. Lay the lemon slices onto each fillet
4. Slip the tray into the oven and bake until the salmon is just cooked
5. Meanwhile, prepare the potatoes: place the potatoes in a large saucepan, sprinkle with a generous dose of salt, and cover with water. Cover, and place over a medium-high heat and allow the water to come to a boil. Once the water is boiling, partially remove the lid and allow the potatoes to simmer until soft

Nutritional information

- ***Calories:*** 428
- ***Fat:*** 23.5 grams
- ***Protein:*** 27.9 grams
- ***Total carbs:*** 29 grams
- ***Net carbs:*** 29 grams

Simple Grilled Octopus with Garlic Butter

This is an easy way to prepare octopus, even for total beginners! We serve it with garlic butter, lemon, and herbs. A great serving suggestion is to serve with asparagus or a simple, fresh salad.

Servings: 4

Time: approximately 2 hours

Ingredients

- 3 lbs fresh octopus (any size you can source)
- 4 Tbsp butter, melted
- 2 Tbsp olive oil
- 5 garlic cloves, finely chopped
- ⅓ cup each of fresh parsley and fresh coriander/cilantro, finely chopped
- Salt and pepper

Method

1. Place the octopus into a large pot of boiling, salted water and leave to boil for about 40 minutes
2. Drain and rinse the cooked octopus
3. In a large bowl, toss together the octopus, garlic, butter, and olive oil and leave to infuse for about 30 minutes
4. Place a griddle pan over a high heat
5. Cut each octopus tentacle lengthways, but don't fully separate
6. Place the octopus onto the hot griddle pan and cook on both sides until slightly charred
7. Serve with a scattering of fresh herbs

Nutritional information

- **Calories:** 445
- **Fat:** 21.3 grams
- **Protein:** 51 grams
- **Total carbs:** 8.7 grams
- **Net carbs:** 8.6 grams

Seafood Stew

A classic, rustic stew featuring mussels, prawns, and fish. We flavor our stew with garlic, tomatoes, onions, and fish sauce. A steaming-hot, comforting bowl of nutrients and the flavor of the Mediterranean Sea.

Servings: 5

Time: approximately 45 minutes

Ingredients

- 2 Tbsp olive oil
- 2 large onions, finely chopped
- 10 garlic cloves, finely chopped
- 3 Tbsp tomato paste
- 1 cup dry white wine
- 5 cups fish or chicken stock
- 2 tsp fish sauce
- 2 cups canned chopped tomatoes
- 10 oz fish, cubed
- 1 lb mussels
- 1 lb prawns
- Salt and pepper
- Fresh parsley

Method

1. Add the olive oil to a very large saucepan or stockpot over a medium-high heat
2. Add the onions and garlic and stir as they soften
3. Add the tomato paste and stir as it melts into the onions and garlic for a minute or two
4. Add the wine and allow the alcohol to burn off for a few minutes, and allow the liquid to reduce
5. Add the stock, fish sauce, and tomatoes and allow the mixture to reach simmering point
6. Season the soup with salt and pepper, taste, and adjust the seasoning as needed

7. Add the fish and cook for 2 minutes, add the prawns and cook for 2 minutes, then add the mussels and cook for 2 minutes

8. Taste and add more seasoning as required

9. Serve piping hot, with fresh parsley scattered over the top!

Nutritional information

- ***Calories:*** 689
- ***Fat:*** 17 grams
- ***Protein:*** 87.4 grams
- ***Total carbs:*** 22 grams
- ***Net carbs:*** 19.7 grams

Weekend Pasta with Anchovies, Lemon, and Chili

I call this "weekend pasta" because it's easy, tasty and comforting, and requires little effort and no trips to the store! As long as you've got dried pasta, anchovies, and a lemon lying around, you can make this tasty dish.

Servings: 2

Time: approximately 20 minutes

Ingredients

- 8 oz dried pasta (any shape!)
- 1 Tbsp olive oil
- 6 anchovies (the kind in oil)
- Juice of 1 lemon
- 1 fresh red chili, finely chopped, or 2 tsp dried chili flakes
- Salt and pepper
- Fresh parsley
- Freshly grated parmesan cheese

Method

1. Place a saucepan of very salty water over a high heat (it should be salty like the Mediterranean Ocean!)
2. Add the pasta to the boiling water
3. As the pasta cooks, prepare the sauce: place the olive oil into a pan over a medium heat. Add the anchovies and uses a wooden spoon to break them up. Allow them to cook and "melt". Add the lemon juice, chili, salt and pepper
4. Drain the pasta (reserve a little of the pasta water) and add it to the pan with the anchovies, quickly toss with a little pasta water to make sure it's silky and shiny (not claggy!)
5. Taste the pasta and add more seasoning if need be
6. Serve with lots of fresh parsley and parmesan cheese

Nutritional information

- ***Calories:*** 589
- ***Fat:*** 16.2 grams

- ***Protein:*** 25.3 grams
- ***Total carbs:*** 84.3 grams
- ***Net carbs:*** 80.8 grams

Crab Salad Cups

This recipe is an excellent way to make the most of crab meat. We fill lettuce cups with crab, avocado, cucumber, radish, lime juice, and chili. Enjoy these for a light meal or serve them as a starter for a Mediterranean diet dinner party!

Servings: 4

Time: approximately 20 minutes

Ingredients

- 12 cos lettuce leaves
- 2 lb fresh, cooked crab meat, cut into small pieces (try to match the size of the vegetables)
- 2 avocados, cubed
- 2 cups sliced cucumber
- 1 cup sliced radish

Dressing:

- Juice of 2 lemons
- 2 Tbsp olive oil
- 1 fresh red chili, finely chopped
- Salt and pepper
- ½ cup finely chopped coriander/cilantro

Method

1. Lay out your cos lettuce leaves/cups onto a board
2. In a bowl, combine the crab meat, avocados, cucumber, and radish
3. Add the dressing ingredients to the bowl with the crab and veggies and gently toss to combine
4. Taste the crab and veggie mixture and add more lime, chili, or salt as required
5. Divide the crab mixture between the cups
6. Serve right away to preserve the freshness of the lettuce!

Nutritional information

- **Calories:** 361
- **Fat:** 21.9 grams

- ***Protein:*** 34.4 grams
- ***Total carbs:*** 11.7 grams
- ***Net carbs:*** 5.3 grams

Mussels with Tomatoes and Garlic

If you've got fresh mussels to use up, this is a wonderful way to do so! We make a rich, tasty, tomato-based broth in which we cook the mussels. You can serve this alone, or with fresh pasta.

Servings: 4

Time: approximately 40 minutes

Ingredients

- 4 Tbsp olive oil
- 8 garlic cloves, finely chopped
- 1 onion, finely chopped
- 4 cups chopped canned tomatoes
- 2 Tbsp balsamic vinegar
- 4 lbs fresh mussels, debearded and scrubbed
- Salt and pepper
- Large handful of fresh parsley, finely chopped

Method

1. Add the olive oil to a large sauté pan over a medium-high heat
2. Add the garlic and onions and stir as they become soft and fragrant
3. Add the tomatoes and vinegar and allow to simmer for about 5 minutes
4. Add the mussels, cover the pot, and cook for about 3 minutes, giving the pan a good shake here and there to ensure nothing is sticking
5. Throw away any unopened mussels
6. Season with salt and pepper, and serve with fresh parsley

Nutritional information

- **Calories:** 385
- **Fat:** 21.4 grams
- **Protein:** 26.5 grams
- **Total carbs:** 23.9 grams
- **Net carbs:** 20.9 grams

Fresh Fish Puttanesca Salad with Couscous

This salad is a take on the popular dish pasta puttanesca, made with olives, capers, tomatoes, and anchovies. This salad features fresh white fish, fresh tomatoes, briny black olives, capers, and dried chili flakes. You can of course, serve it with pasta, but I like to serve it on a bed of buttery couscous!

Servings: 4

Time: approximately 25 minutes

Ingredients

- 1 cup couscous (uncooked)
- 1 Tbsp butter
- Salt and pepper
- 2 Tbsp olive oil
- 1 ½ lbs fresh white fish, cut into even chunks
- 1 Tbsp dried chili flakes
- Salt and pepper
- ½ cup roughly chopped fresh basil
- 4 tomatoes, chopped
- 25 black olives, pits removed, roughly chopped
- 4 Tbsp capers

Method

1. In a bowl, add the couscous, butter, salt and pepper. Pour over 1 cup of boiling water, cover, and leave as you prepare the rest of the dish
2. Add the olive oil to a pan over a medium heat
3. Add the fish and cook on each side until golden and just cooked through
4. Add the chili pepper and season with salt and pepper, remove from the heat
5. Use a fork to fluff the couscous and distribute the butter throughout
6. Divide the couscous between four serving bowls
7. In a bow, gently combine the fish, basil, tomatoes, olives, and capers
8. Divide the fish mixture between the four bowl and spoon over the piles of fluffy couscous

9. Serve with an extra drizzle of olive oil!

Nutritional information

- **Calories:** 464
- **Fat:** 14.5 grams
- **Protein:** 40 grams
- **Total carbs:** 44.4 grams
- **Net carbs:** 40.1 grams

Pan-Fried Scallops with Fresh Fennel Salad

Scallops are soft, creamy, and decadent. They're a sure way to impress a date or dinner party guests! We serve these with a fresh and crispy fennel salad.

Servings: 4

Time: approximately 30 minutes

Ingredients

- 16 fresh scallops
- 2 Tbsp olive oil
- 2 Tbsp butter
- Salt and pepper
- Juice of 1 lemon
- 4 cups finely sliced fresh fennel bulb
- 1 cup finely sliced celery
- ¾ cup chopped almonds, gently toasted until light golden
- Juice of 1 orange
- 2 Tbsp olive oil
- ½ cup chopped fresh basil
- ⅓ cup chopped fresh mint
- Salt and pepper

Method

1. Prep the salad first: simply toss together the ingredients, taste, and add more seasoning, oil, herbs, or orange juice as needed
2. Place a frying pan over a medium heat (preferably a non-stick pan!)
3. Add the olive oil and butter to the pan and allow to melt
4. Pat the scallops dry with a paper towel and add them to the hot pan (do this in batches if you need to)
5. Sprinkle the scallops with salt and pepper while they're in the pan
6. Cook one side for about 3 minutes, then flip and cook the other side until both sides are golden, but be careful not to overcook them!

7. Squeeze the lemon over the scallops and remove from the heat
8. Serve the scallops on top of a pile of fresh, crunchy salad

Nutritional information

- **Calories:** 361
- **Fat:** 32.5 grams
- **Protein:** 16.4 grams
- **Total carbs:** 11.1 grams
- **Net carbs:** 7.5 grams

Clams with Creamy Polenta

If you can source fresh clams, you absolutely have to make this rich and decadent meal! We steam the clams with a creamy, garlicky, white wine sauce and serve them with creamy polenta. Restaurant-quality food in the comfort of home.

Servings: 4

Time: approximately 30 minutes

Ingredients

- 1 Tbsp olive oil
- 3 Tbsp butter
- 8 garlic cloves, finely chopped
- 3 lbs fresh clams
- 1 cup dry white wine
- 1 cup water or chicken stock
- Juice of 1 lemon
- ¾ cup full-fat, heavy cream
- Salt and pepper
- Fresh parsley
- 1 cup instant polenta
- 4 cups water
- 1 Tbsp butter
- ½ cup full-fat milk
- ½ cup grated parmesan
- Salt and pepper

Method

1. Add the olive oil, butter, and garlic into a large sauté pan over a medium heat
2. Stir as the butter and olive oil melt together and the garlic becomes fragrant
3. Add the clams and stir to coat in butter
4. Add the wine and allow to reduce for about 5 minutes

5. Add the water or stock and allow everything to come to a simmer so that the clams can open up
6. Once the clams have opened, add the lemon juice, cream, salt, pepper, and parsley and stir to combine
7. To make the polenta: bring the water to a rolling boil and add the polenta, whisking the whole time. Turn the heat down and keep whisking as the polenta thickens. Add the butter and whisk as it melts into the polenta. Whisk in the milk, parmesan, salt, and pepper
8. Serve the clams and sauce spooned over the creamy polenta…blissful!

Nutritional information

- **Calories:** 983
- **Fat:** 63.3 grams
- **Protein:** 71.7 grams
- **Total carbs:** 46.6 grams
- **Net carbs:** 45.5 grams

Legumes and Vegetables

This is the largest section in this book, as vegetables and legumes are the most important building blocks of the Mediterranean diet. The great thing is that you can mix and match most of the recipes in this book. For example, you may like to create a salad from this section, and pair it with a meat or poultry dish for one of your allocated "meat nights", or simply enjoy the dish alone. Whenever you can, source fresh, local produce. However, this isn't always easy depending on your location and the changing conditions of the seasons. For this reason, it's completely okay to use frozen or imported produce in a pinch! What's more, canned beans, lentils, and chickpeas are also completely permitted, encouraged, in fact! In this section, you will find refreshing salads, comforting soups and stews, decadent risottos, and many more vegetarian delights.

Pearl Barley, Citrus, and Broccoli Salad

Pearl barley is a filling, nutritious, and versatile grain which can be thrown into anything from soups to stews to salads. This recipe combines pearl barley with fresh orange, crunchy broccoli, nuts, and a little feta cheese for salty "bite"

Servings: 4

Time: approximately 45 minutes

Ingredients

- 1 ½ cups pearl barley
- 4 ¼ cups water
- Salt
- 2 oranges, peeled and chopped
- 1 medium-large head of broccoli, cut into florets
- 3 oz feta cheese, crumbled
- ⅓ cup chopped almonds, gently toasted
- ⅓ cup chopped hazelnuts, gently toasted
- ½ cup finely chopped parsley
- 3 Tbsp olive oil
- Salt and pepper

Method

1. Place the barley, water, and salt into a saucepan over a medium heat, cover, and bring to boiling point
2. Reduce to a simmer, and partially remove the cover
3. Keep an eye on the barley and add a dash of water if it appears to be drying out
4. When the barley is plump and there is no liquid left, remove the pot from the heat and allow the barley to cool a little
5. Place a steamer over a saucepan of shallow, boiling water, add the broccoli to the steamer, cover, and cook until the broccoli is just cooked but still crunchy and vibrant in color
6. Combine the pearl barley, broccoli, feta, almonds, hazelnuts, parsley, olive oil, salt and pepper in a salad bowl and toss to combine

Nutritional information

- ***Calories:*** 569
- ***Fat:*** 28.2 grams
- ***Protein:*** 19.1 grams
- ***Total carbs:*** 80 grams
- ***Net carbs:*** 60 grams

Creamy Rice Risotto with Mushrooms and Thyme

It's hard to imagine rice risotto being met with anything but pure delight! This risotto features earthy, rich mushrooms, fragrant thyme, and parmesan cheese, of course. This is a comforting dish ideal for cold, Wintery weekend nights.

Servings: 4

Time: approximately 35 minutes

Ingredients

- 2 Tbsp olive oil
- 1 onion, finely chopped
- 4 garlic cloves, finely chopped
- 13 oz Arborio rice
- 4 cups sliced mushrooms (use any type!)
- ½ cup dry white wine
- 2 Tbsp thyme leaves, finely chopped
- 6 ½ cups vegetable or chicken stock
- 3 Tbsp butter
- ½ cup grated parmesan cheese
- Salt and pepper

Method

1. Place the stock into a saucepan over a medium heat, it shouldn't boil, but should be hot and steaming
2. Add the olive oil to a large sauté pan or pot over a medium heat
3. Add the onion and garlic and stir as they soften and become fragrant, about 3 minutes
4. Add the rice and stir to coat in olive oil, allow the rice to become acquainted with the flavor of the onion and garlic, about 3 minutes
5. Add the mushrooms and stir as they soften for about 3 minutes
6. Add the wine and stir to deglaze the corners of the pan, allow it to reduce for about 3 minutes
7. Add the thyme leaves and stir

8. Add a dash of hot stock, stir, and allow it to be absorbed into the rice. Repeat this process, adding dashes of hot stock, stirring, and allowing to absorb, until all of the stock has been used up and the risotto is creamy

9. Stir the butter, parmesan, salt and pepper into the risotto, cover, and leave for at least 5 minutes. This step is crucial for a creamy risotto! The butter and cheese melt, and the starches from the rice have time to relax and create a silky, rich consistency

10. Serve with a little extra sprinkle of grated parmesan and a few thyme leaves!

Nutritional information

- *Calories:* 608
- *Fat:* 19.4 grams
- *Protein:* 23.2 grams
- *Total carbs:* 80.3 grams
- *Net carbs:* 79.8 grams

Herbed Polenta with Roasted Veggies

Instant polenta is an excellent staple ingredient to keep in your cupboard. It's incredibly easy and fast to prepare, and can be used as a base for many dishes. This dish is a collection of veggies, roasted to soft perfection, and piled on top of herby, creamy polenta

Servings: 4

Time: approximately 1 hour

Ingredients

- 3 large agria potatoes (or any roasting variety you have), cut into chunks
- 3 large carrots, cut into chunks
- 2 leeks, white parts cut into chunks
- 2 red bell peppers, sliced
- 2 large zucchini, cut into chunks
- 1 large red onion, cut into chunks
- 3 Tbsp olive oil
- Salt and pepper
- 1 cup instant polenta
- 4 cups water
- 1 Tbsp butter
- ½ cup full-fat milk
- ½ cup grated parmesan
- 3 Tbsp each finely chopped thyme, parsley, mint, and oregano
- Salt and pepper

Method

1. Preheat the oven to 400 degrees Fahrenheit and have a roasting pan waiting by
2. Pile the veggies into the pan, pour over the olive oil, sprinkle over the salt and pepper, and rub the veggies to ensure each piece is coated in oil and seasoning
3. Place the tray in the oven and roast for about 40 minutes or until the veggies are golden and tender. Toss or turn the veggies halfway through
4. Prepare the polenta 5 minutes before you take the veggies out of the oven: pour the water into a saucepan with a generous dash of salt, and place over a medium-high heat until the

water is just starting to boil. Whisk continuously as you pour the polenta into the water, keep whisking until the polenta is thick and creamy, it won't take long! Add the butter, parmesan, herbs, salt and pepper and stir to combine

5. Divide the polenta between 4 serving plates and pile the veggies on top

Nutritional information

- **Calories:** 740
- **Fat:** 28.8 grams
- **Protein:** 29 grams
- **Total carbs:** 93.8 grams
- **Net carbs:** 84.3 grams

Brown Rice, Feta, Fresh Pea, and Mint Salad

Brown rice is a nutty, chewy, easy staple which adds bulk and fiber to any dish. It's excellent when served cold, as the foundation of a salad. This salad features peas, mint, and feta cheese

Servings: 4

Time: approximately 40 minutes

Ingredients

- 2 cups brown rice
- 2 ¾ cups water
- Salt
- 5 oz feta cheese, crumbled
- 2 cups fresh or frozen peas, boiled until just cooked but still robust and vibrant
- ½ cup chopped fresh mint
- 2 Tbsp olive oil
- Salt and pepper

Method

1. Place the brown rice, water, and salt into a saucepan over a medium heat, cover, and bring to boiling point. Turn the heat down and allow to cook until the water has dissolved and the rice is soft yet chewy. Leave to cool completely
2. Add the feta, peas, mint, olive oil, salt, and pepper to a salad bowl with the cooled rice and toss to combine
3. Serve!

Nutritional information

- **Calories:** 613
- **Fat:** 18.2 grams
- **Protein:** 21 grams
- **Total carbs:** 95.4 grams
- **Net carbs:** 85.4 grams

Whole Grain Pita Bread Stuffed with Olives, Tomatoes, and Chickpeas

Whole-grain pita pockets are perfect little parcels for stuffing with tasty, Med-inspired fillings. These pita pockets are filled with a nutrient-dense mixture of olives, chickpeas, and tomatoes

Servings: 2

Time: approximately 20 minutes

Ingredients

- 2 wholegrain pita pockets
- 2 Tbsp olive oil
- 2 garlic cloves, finely chopped
- 1 small onion, finely chopped
- ½ tsp cumin
- 10 black olives, stones removed, roughly chopped
- 2 cups cooked chickpeas (canned is fine!)
- Salt and pepper

Method

1. Slice open the pita pockets and have them waiting by
2. Add the olive oil to a pan over a medium heat
3. Add the garlic, onion, and turmeric to the hot pan and stir as the onions soften and the cumin is fragrant
4. Add the olives, chickpeas, salt and pepper and toss everything together and the chickpeas become golden
5. Remove the pan from the heat and use your wooden spoon to roughly mash the chickpeas so that some are intact and some are crushed
6. Heat your pita pockets in the microwave, in the oven, or on a clean pan on the stove
7. Fill them with your chickpea mixture and devour!

Nutritional information

- **Calories:** 509
- **Fat:** 19 grams

- ***Protein:*** 15.7 grams
- ***Total carbs:*** 72 grams
- ***Net carbs:*** 59.4 grams

Beetroot and Goat Cheese Salad with Toasted Barley

Beetroot and goat cheese go together so harmoniously. We pair them together in this nutty salad featuring barley as the base.

Servings: 4

Time: approximately 40 minutes

Ingredients

- 1 ½ cups pearl barley
- 4 ½ cups water
- Salt
- 1 Tbsp olive oil
- 2 large fresh beets, peeled and cut into chunks
- 1 Tbsp olive oil
- Fresh thyme
- 4 oz goat cheese, crumbled
- 6 Tbsp pumpkin seeds, lightly toasted
- 4 cups baby spinach leaves, roughly chopped
- Salt and pepper
- Juice of 1 lemon

Method

1. Preheat the oven to 400 degrees Fahrenheit and line a baking tray with baking paper
2. Lay the beets onto the tray, rub with olive oil, and sprinkle with salt, thyme leaves, and pepper and place into the oven to roast for about 30 minutes or until soft, turning halfway through
3. Place the barley, water, and salt into a saucepan over a medium heat, cover, and bring to boiling point. Reduce the heat and allow the barley to simmer until there's no liquid left, and the barley is chewy
4. Push the beets aside on the baking tray and spread the cooked barley onto the tray and slip into the oven to toast for about 15 minutes (if you're worried about overcooking the beets you can transfer them into a salad bowl at this point)

5. In a salad bowl, toss together the beets, barley, goat cheese, spinach, pumpkin seeds, salt, pepper, and lemon juice
6. Serve warm or cold

Nutritional information

- ***Calories:*** 506
- ***Fat:*** 21.7 grams
- ***Protein:*** 18.4 grams
- ***Total carbs:*** 63.8 grams
- ***Net carbs:*** 50 grams

Roasted Carrots with Walnuts and Cannellini Beans

When carrots are roasted in the oven, they become irresistibly soft and sweet. We add walnuts, a little honey, and cannellini beans to this simple tray-bake dish.

Servings: 4

Time: approximately 45 minutes

Ingredients

- 4 large carrots, peeled and cut into batons
- 1 cup walnuts
- 1 Tbsp honey
- 2 Tbsp olive oil
- 2 cups canned cannellini beans (2 cups when drained)
- 1 fresh thyme sprig
- Salt and pepper

Method

1. Preheat the oven to 400 degrees Fahrenheit and line a baking tray or roasting pan with baking paper
2. Lay the carrots and walnuts onto the lined tray or pan
3. Drizzle the honey and olive oil over the carrots and walnuts and give everything a rub to make sure each piece is coated
4. Scatter the beans onto the tray and nestle into the carrots and walnuts
5. Nestle the thyme into the beans and sprinkle everything with salt and pepper
6. Pop the tray into the oven and roast for about 40 minutes or until the carrots are soft and tender

Nutritional information

- **Calories:** 385
- **Fat:** 26.9 grams
- **Protein:** 11.7 grams
- **Total carbs:** 33.2 grams
- **Net carbs:** 22.2 grams

Rustic White Bean Soup

White bean soup is so easy to make, but results in a velvety, smooth, creamy soup to impress absolutely anyone! Serve with a piece of crusty, whole grain bread and a little dish of olive oil for dipping. Note that this recipe contains bacon!

Servings: 4

Time: approximately 35 minutes

Ingredients

- 10 rashers of streaky bacon, cut into small pieces
- 2 onions, finely chopped
- 10 garlic cloves, finely chopped
- 3 large carrots, peeled and roughly chopped
- 3 celery sticks, roughly chopped
- ½ cup white wine
- 4 cups chicken or vegetable stock
- 30 oz canned cannellini beans (don't drain)
- 1 bay leaf
- 1 fresh rosemary sprig
- 1 thyme sprig
- Salt and pepper
- ½ cup heavy cream (can omit this if you're watching calories)
- ½ cup grated parmesan cheese

Method

1. Place a stock pot or large saucepan over a medium-high heat
2. Add the bacon and stir as it sizzles and the fat renders
3. Add the onions, garlic, carrots, and celery and stir as they soften, about 5 minutes
4. Add the wine and allow to reduce for 2 minutes
5. Add the stock, beans, bay leaf, rosemary, thyme, salt, and pepper, cover the pot and simmer for about 20 minutes
6. Use a stick blender to blend the soup gently, so that it still has a little texture

7. Stir in the cream and parmesan into the soup
8. Serve hot!

Nutritional information

- **Calories:** 567
- **Fat:** 27.8 grams
- **Protein:** 26.7 grams
- **Total carbs:** 51 grams
- **Net carbs:** 34.4 grams

Simple Weeknight Pasta with Olives, Tomatoes, and Ricotta

We all need an easy pasta recipe up our sleeve to pull out on a busy, tired evening. This pasta features fresh tomatoes, olives, and creamy ricotta cheese. You can use any pasta shape you have, but I like to use penne

Servings: 4

Time: approximately 30 minutes

Ingredients

- 16 oz dried penne pasta
- 4 large, fresh tomatoes, roughly chopped
- 20 black olives, stones removed, roughly chopped
- 8 oz full-fat ricotta cheese
- 1 tsp dried chili flakes
- Salt and pepper
- 2 Tbsp olive oil
- Fresh basil

Method

1. Place a saucepan of very salty water over a high heat, cover, and bring to boiling point
2. Add the pasta and leave to boil, uncovered
3. When the pasta is cooked, drain, but reserve a little of the pasta water in the pan
4. Add the tomatoes, olives, chili flakes, olive oil, salt, and pepper to the pan and place it over a medium heat and stir to break up the tomatoes and allow them to form a sauce with the oil and pasta water
5. Stir the ricotta into the pasta just before serving
6. Serve with a scattering of fresh basil

Nutritional information

- **Calories:** 374
- **Fat:** 16.3 grams
- **Protein:** 13.6 grams
- **Total carbs:** 42.1 grams

- ***Net carbs:*** 37 grams

Quinoa Risotto

Risotto doesn't always need to be made with rice! It can be made with quinoa for a nutrient-dense, rich, and unique meal

Servings: 4

Time: approximately 45 minutes

Ingredients

- 2 Tbsp olive oil
- 1 onion, finely chopped
- 5 garlic cloves, finely chopped
- 1 ½ cups dry quinoa, thoroughly rinsed
- ½ cup dry white wine
- 5 cups chicken or vegetable stock
- 2 Tbsp butter
- ¾ cup grated parmesan cheese
- Salt and pepper

Method

1. Pour the stock into a saucepan over a medium heat, it shouldn't boil but should be steaming
2. Add the olive oil to a deep-sided sauté pan over a medium heat
3. Add the onion and garlic and stir as they soften
4. Add the quinoa and stir to combine with the onions and garlic, keep stirring for about 2 minutes
5. Add the wine, stir, and allow it to reduce for a couple of minutes
6. Add a little of the hot stock to the quinoa, stir, and allow it to soak into the quinoa. Repeat this process until all of the stock has been used up and the quinoa is creamy
7. Stir the butter and parmesan into the risotto, cover, and leave to sit for 5 minutes
8. Stir the risotto again, and serve with an extra grating of parmesan

Nutritional information

- ***Calories:*** 466

- ***Fat:*** 21.5 grams
- ***Protein:*** 16.7 grams
- ***Total carbs:*** 47.1 grams
- ***Net carbs:*** 42 grams

Artichokes Provencal

Artichokes Provencal is a simple and fast way to make the most of in-season artichokes. We pile together artichokes, tomatoes, onions, garlic, and basil with a little wine and lemon

Servings: 4

Time: approximately 20 minutes

Ingredients

- 1 Tbsp olive oil
- 1 onion, roughly chopped
- 4 garlic cloves, finely chopped
- ½ cup dry white wine
- 4 tomatoes, chopped
- 10 oz artichoke hearts, quartered
- 1 lemon, quartered
- Salt and pepper
- Fresh basil, roughly chopped or torn

Method

1. Add the olive oil to a large sauté pan over a medium-high heat
2. Add the onions and garlic and stir as they soften, about 5 minutes
3. Add the wine and allow to reduce for a few minutes
4. Add the artichokes, tomatoes, salt, pepper, and lemon quarters, cover, and cook for about 5-8 minutes or until the artichokes are tender
5. Serve with fresh basil

Nutritional information

- **Calories:** 159
- **Fat:** 7 grams
- **Protein:** 2.8 grams
- **Total carbs:** 15.5 grams
- **Net carbs:** 13.5 grams

Eggplant and Potato Traybake with Yogurt Dressing

This traybake features comforting potatoes, soft eggplant, sweet red onion, and a tangy yogurt dressing

Servings: 5

Time: approximately 35 minutes

Ingredients

- 2 large eggplants, cut into even chunks
- 4 large potatoes, cut into even chunks
- 2 red onions, cut into even chunks
- 4 Tbsp olive oil
- Salt and pepper
- ½ cup plain Greek yogurt
- Juice of ½ lemon
- 2 Tbsp finely chopped fresh mint
- Salt and pepper

Method

1. Preheat the oven to 400 degrees Fahrenheit and line a baking tray with baking paper
2. Lay the eggplant, potatoes, and onion onto the tray and rub with olive oil salt and pepper
3. Roast the veggies for about 30 minutes or until soft and golden (depending on your oven, you may have to roast them for longer), give them a toss halfway through
4. Combine the yogurt, lemon juice, mint, salt and pepper
5. Serve the roasted veggies with the yogurt sauce on the side

Nutritional information

- **Calories:** 270
- **Fat:** 12.5 grams
- **Protein:** 5.4 grams
- **Total carbs:** 38.3 grams
- **Net carbs:** 29.3 grams

Bulgur and Roasted Bell Pepper Salad

Bulgur wheat is a fantastic alternative to rice, couscous or quinoa, especially when it is tossed with seasonal vegetables and served as a "bowl food" style salad. This recipe combines toasted and cooked bulgur with roasted bell pepper

Servings: 4

Time: approximately 40 minutes

Ingredients

- 3 large red bell peppers, seeds removed, sliced
- 1 red onion, sliced
- 2 Tbsp olive oil
- Salt and pepper
- 2 Tbsp butter
- 1 Tbsp olive oil
- 2 cups bulgur (dry)
- 4 cups water
- Salt

Method

1. Preheat the oven to 400 degrees Fahrenheit and line a baking tray with baking paper
2. Spread the bell pepper and onion over the tray and rub with olive oil, salt and pepper
3. Roast the bell pepper and onion for about 30 minutes, tossing once, until very soft and slightly charred and gooey
4. Add the butter and oil in a sauté pan over a medium heat
5. When the butter and oil are hot, add the dry bulgur and stir as it toasts, about 2 minutes
6. Add the water and salt to the pan, cover, and cook until the water has evaporated and the bulgur is fluffy and tender
7. Add the roasted bell pepper and onion to the bulgur, toss, and serve

Serving suggestions: fresh basil or mint and a side of lemony Greek yogurt

Nutritional information

- ***Calories:*** 428
- ***Fat:*** 17 grams
- ***Protein:*** 10 grams
- ***Total carbs:*** 63 grams
- ***Net carbs:*** 51 grams

Brown Lentil Salad with Grilled Halloumi

If I'm at a cafe or restaurant and there's halloumi on the menu? I'm ordering it! This dish involves brown lentils (canned for ease!) tossed with lemon, cucumber, and pine nuts, with golden strips of grilled halloumi on top

Servings: 4

Time: approximately 30 minutes

Ingredients

- 2 cans brown lentils (rinsed and drained)
- Juice and zest of 1 lemon
- 2 cups chopped cucumber (I leave the seeds in!)
- ½ cup toasted pine nuts (use almonds or cashews if pine nuts are too expensive in your region)
- 2 Tbsp olive oil
- 14 oz halloumi cheese, cut into strips

Method

1. Preheat the oven to 450 degrees Fahrenheit and line a baking tray with baking paper
2. In a large salad bowl, toss together the lentils, lemon, cucumber, pine nuts, and olive oil, set aside or refrigerate as you cook the halloumi
3. Place the halloumi slices onto the lined tray and cook in the upper third of the oven for about 12 minutes, turn the slices over, and cook until the other side is golden
4. Serve the salad with halloumi slices on top

Nutritional information

- ***Calories:*** 665
- ***Fat:*** 43.7 grams
- ***Protein:*** 38 grams
- ***Total carbs:*** 36.7 grams
- ***Net carbs:*** 27.5 grams

Israeli Couscous with Zucchini, Peas, and Feta

Israeli couscous consists of chewy, orb-like morsels which resemble pasta in flavor and texture. You can toss almost anything with Israeli couscous, from fish to roasted veggies. For this recipe, we are tossing it with peas, feta, and roasted zucchini

Servings: 4

Time: approximately 30 minutes

Ingredients

- 2 large zucchini, cut into rounds
- 2 Tbsp olive oil
- Salt and pepper
- Rosemary sprig
- 1 lemon, quartered
- 1 Tbsp olive oil
- 1 Tbsp butter
- 4 garlic cloves, roughly chopped
- 2 cups israeli couscous (dry)
- 4 cups chicken or vegetable stock
- Salt and pepper
- 2 cups frozen peas, cooked (microwave, steam, or boil)
- 4 oz feta cheese, crumbled

Method

1. Preheat the oven to 400 degrees Fahrenheit and line a baking tray with baking paper
2. Lay the zucchini rounds onto the tray, rub with olive oil, salt, and pepper. Nestle the rosemary and lemon quarters into the zucchini and slip into the oven to roast for about 30 minutes
3. While the zucchini is cooking, prepare the couscous: add the olive oil, butter, and garlic into a deep-sided sauté pan over a medium heat and allow the butter to melt and become frothy. Add the Israeli couscous, toss in the oil and butter, and toast for about 5 minutes. Add the stock, cover, and leave to cook until the stock has evaporated and the couscous is tender
4. Add the zucchini, peas, and feta to the pan with the couscous. Take the roasted lemon quarters and squeeze the gooey flesh and juices into the couscous and toss to combine

5. Serve warm or cold!

Nutritional information

- ***Calories:*** 610
- ***Fat:*** 20 grams
- ***Protein:*** 23.6 grams
- ***Total carbs:*** 86.5 grams
- ***Net carbs:*** 76.4 grams

Fresh Watermelon and Goat Cheese Salad

If there's one salad you must include on your Summertime dinner table, it's this one. Sweet, juicy watermelon, fresh mint, and tangy goat cheese make an idyllic salad. We add toasted pistachio nuts for extra color and texture

Servings: 4

Time: approximately 15 minutes

Ingredients

- 6 cups watermelon cubes
- ½ cup finely sliced fresh mint
- 5 oz goat cheese, crumbled
- ½ cup chopped pistachios, toasted
- 2 Tbsp olive oil
- Juice of ½ lime
- Salt and pepper

Method

1. Gently toss together all ingredients in a salad bowl and ensure the olive oil and lime juice is evenly distributed
2. Serve chilled

Nutritional information

- **Calories:** 310
- **Fat:** 21.5 grams
- **Protein:** 11.1 grams
- **Total carbs:** 22 grams
- **Net carbs:** 19.5 grams

Broccoli and Lentil Cakes with Avocado

Broccoli lends itself so wonderfully to a wide range of dishes, even patties! These patties are made with broccoli, lentils, egg, herbs, and a little grated mozzarella. We serve them in pita pockets with ripe avocado

Servings: 4

Time: approximately 30 minutes

Ingredients

- 4 cups broccoli that has been blitzed in the food processor until it is the size of rice
- 2 cups canned brown lentils, drained
- 2 eggs
- ½ cup plain flour
- ¾ cup grated mozzarella cheese
- 2 Tbsp each finely chopped mint and parsley
- Salt and pepper
- Olive oil for frying
- 1 avocado, sliced
- 4 pita pockets

Method

1. Place the blitzed broccoli into a microwave-safe bowl, cover, and cook in the microwave for about 3 minutes or until the broccoli is just starting to soften
2. Place the broccoli, lentils, eggs, flour, mozzarella, herbs, salt, and pepper into a food processor and pulse until a batter forms
3. Drizzle a little olive oil into a non-stick pan over a medium-high heat
4. Take spoonfuls of the broccoli mixture and drop them onto the hot pan, cook for a couple of minutes, turn, then cook the other side until golden
5. Slice open your pita pockets, heat (the toaster works just fine!) and slip a couple of avocado slices into each one, then add a few patties (depending on the size of them, just add as many as you need to neatly fill the pita)
6. Serve!

Serving suggestion: a little Greek yogurt spread into the pita would be lovely!

Nutritional information

- **Calories:** 584
- **Fat:** 21.1 grams
- **Protein:** 31 grams
- **Total carbs:** 76.6 grams
- **Net carbs:** 63.1 grams

Roasted Sweet Potatoes with Pomegranates and Red Onion

Plain roasted sweet potatoes are lovely, sure, but they're unbelievable when served with pomegranate arils, red onion, and pumpkin seeds

Servings: 4

Time: approximately 40 minutes

Ingredients

- 2 lbs sweet potatoes, cut into even chunks
- 2 Tbsp olive oil
- Salt and pepper
- 6 Tbsp pumpkin seeds
- ½ red onion, finely chopped
- 2 pomegranates

Method

1. Preheat the oven to 400 degrees Fahrenheit and line a baking tray with baking paper
2. Spread the sweet potatoes over the lined tray, and rub with olive oil, salt, and pepper
3. Slip the tray into the preheated oven and roast the sweet potatoes for about 20 minutes, turn them over, and add the pumpkin seeds (if we add them too soon they will burn, so we add them halfway through!) and roast until the sweet potatoes are golden and soft
4. Transfer the sweet potatoes and pumpkin seeds to a large salad bowl and add the red onion
5. Cut the pomegranates in half, hold the cut side over splayed fingers, and tap the back of the fruit so that the arils fall into the bowl but the white, pithy parts are caught in your hands. Make sure you get a decent amount of juice into the bowl, as it acts as a sweet dressing!
6. Serve warm or cold

Nutritional information

- ***Calories:*** 472
- ***Fat:*** 16.3 grams
- ***Protein:*** 11.6 grams
- ***Total carbs:*** 76.6 grams
- ***Net carbs:*** 62 grams

Honeyed Eggplant

When eggplant is roasted in the oven after being coated in olive oil, honey, and sesame seeds, it takes on the most amazing flavor and texture. It can be served as part of a Mediterranean dinner party, amongst an array of small plates, dips, and large salads

Servings: 4

Time: approximately 35 minutes

Ingredients

- 3 large eggplants, sliced into rounds (remove and discard both ends)
- 4 Tbsp olive oil
- ⅓ cup honey
- Salt and pepper
- 2 Tbsp fresh thyme leaves
- 4 Tbsp sesame seeds

Method

1. Preheat the oven to 400 degrees Fahrenheit and line a baking tray with baking paper
2. Spread the eggplant rounds onto the tray
3. Combine the olive oil, eggplant, salt, pepper, and thyme in a cup and heat for about 15 seconds in the microwave or until the honey has thinned out and you can combine everything to create a cohesive glaze
4. Drizzle the glaze over the eggplant rounds and use a pastry brush to evenly distribute it over both sides of each round
5. Sprinkle the sesame seeds over the glaze and slip the tray into the oven
6. Bake for about 20 minutes, then turn the slices over and cook the other side until golden, soft, and sticky
7. Serve alone, or with crusty bread and a fresh salad

Nutritional information

- **Calories:** 359
- **Fat:** 18.7 grams

- ***Protein:*** 5.7 grams
- ***Total carbs:*** 49.5 grams
- ***Net carbs:*** 36.1 grams

Flatbreads with Roasted Cauliflower, Yogurt, and Asparagus

If you're craving a tasty, filling, and simple dinner on a Friday night, this recipe is perfect. We roast cauliflower and asparagus, then wrap them in a flatbread with yogurt, arugula, and a few spicy chickpeas

Servings: 4

Time: approximately 45 minutes

Ingredients

- 1 medium cauliflower head, cut into florets
- 16 asparagus spears, woody ends removed
- 1 red onion, finely sliced
- 1 cup canned chickpeas, drained
- 3 Tbsp olive oil
- Salt and pepper
- 1 tsp paprika
- 1 tsp ground chili
- 4 flatbreads
- 4 Tbsp Greek yogurt
- 2 cups fresh arugula

Method

1. Preheat the oven to 400 degrees Fahrenheit and line a baking tray with baking paper
2. Spread the cauliflower, asparagus, and chickpeas onto the tray, drizzle with olive oil and sprinkle over the salt, pepper, paprika, and chili
3. Slip the tray into the oven and roast for 20 minutes, give everything a good shake and turn, then cook for a further 10-15 minutes or until everything is golden, toasted, and tender
4. Heat your flatbread, spread yogurt over each one, lay down a bed of arugula, then spoon the roasted veggies and chickpeas over the top

Nutritional information

- **Calories:** 374
- **Fat:** 15 grams

- ***Protein:*** 13.5 grams
- ***Total carbs:*** 49.9 grams
- ***Net carbs:*** 41.1 grams

Mediterranean Spaghetti Squash

Spaghetti squash is a fantastic alternative to pasta, when you feel like going a little lighter on the carbs and starch. We roast the squash until soft, then fill with fresh tomatoes, mozzarella, basil, and olives

Servings: 4

Time: approximately 50 minutes

Ingredients

- 1 medium-large spaghetti squash
- 3 large tomatoes, chopped
- 6 oz fresh mozzarella, roughly torn or sliced
- Large handful of fresh basil leaves
- 10 black olives, stones removed, roughly chopped
- 2 Tbsp olive oil
- Salt and pepper

Method

1. Preheat the oven to 400 degrees Fahrenheit and line a baking tray with baking paper
2. Carefully cut the squash in half, lengthwise and scrape out the seeds
3. Rub the cut sides with olive oil, sprinkle a little salt, and lay cut-side down on your tray
4. Slip the tray into the oven and bake the squash for about 45 minutes or until the flesh is soft
5. Use a fork to fluff the spaghetti squash flesh (gently) and fill each half with tomatoes, mozzarella, basil, olives, and drizzle with olive oil, salt, and pepper (I like to mix everything together, but make sure there's a decent few chunks of mozzarella on top)
6. Place the tray back into the oven for 15 minutes or until the mozzarella is soft and melty, and the tomatoes are soft and soupy
7. Serve hot!

Nutritional information

- **Calories:** 275
- **Fat:** 16.4 grams

- ***Protein:*** 10 grams
- ***Total carbs:*** 24.3 grams
- ***Net carbs:*** 19.5 grams

Cauliflower Rice Med-Style

Blitzed cauliflower can be used for anything from pizza bases to patties. But for this recipe, we are making fried rice! We are flavoring our fried rice with mediterranean-inspired ingredients such as lemon, parsley, almonds, and a secret ingredient for rich flavor...anchovies

Servings: 4

Time: approximately 25 minutes

Ingredients

- 3 anchovies
- 2 Tbsp olive oil
- 1 lemon
- 1 cauliflower head, blitzed in the food processor until it resembles rice
- ½ cup finely chopped parsley
- ½ cup slivered almonds
- Salt and pepper

Method

1. Place the cauliflower rice into a tea towel and squeeze out all of the moisture you can
2. Place a sauté pan over a medium-high heat and add the anchovies and oil
3. Mash the anchovies with a wooden spoon until they disintegrate into the oil
4. Squeeze in the lemon juice (be careful as it may spit)
5. Add the cauliflower rice, parsley, and almonds and toss everything together rapidly
6. Keep stirring as everything toasts and becomes golden
7. Serve hot!

Nutritional information

- **Calories:** 185
- **Fat:** 14.8 grams
- **Protein:** 6.3 grams
- **Total carbs:** 8.3 grams
- **Net carbs:** 3.9 grams

Cauliflower Dough Pizza

Were you waiting patiently for a pizza recipe?! Well, here it is! But this is no ordinary pizza. The base is made from cauliflower, so it's gluten-free (if you use gluten-free flour) and also suits low-carb eaters too. We top our pizza with classic toppings, but you can always improvise and create your own masterpiece!

Servings: makes 2 pizzas, about 4 servings

Time: approximately 45 minutes

Ingredients

- 1 cauliflower head, blitzed in the food processor until fine
- 2 eggs
- ⅓ cup flour
- ½ cup grated parmesan cheese
- Salt and pepper
- 2 Tbsp tomato paste
- 8 oz fresh mozzarella
- 1 cup arugula
- Olive oil

Method

1. Preheat the oven to 400 degrees Fahrenheit and line 2 baking trays with baking paper
2. Place the cauliflower into a tea towel and squeeze out as much liquid as you can
3. Place the squeezed cauliflower into a large bowl and add the eggs, flour, cheese, salt and pepper and stir vigorously until you have a firm dough
4. Press the dough out onto the two trays so that you have two pizza bases
5. Slip the pizza bases into the oven to bake until golden
6. Spread the pre-baked bases with tomato paste and lay the mozzarella over top
7. Bake for a further 10 minutes or until the mozzarella is melted
8. Scatter the arugula over the top and drizzle with olive oil before serving!

Nutritional information

- ***Calories:*** 359
- ***Fat:*** 22.4 grams
- ***Protein:*** 21.3 grams
- ***Total carbs:*** 19.3 grams
- ***Net carbs:*** 15.8 grams

Strawberry and Balsamic Salad

Strawberries and balsamic vinegar are a heavenly match, especially when tossed together in a fresh side salad perfect for any Summer occasion

Servings: 4

Time: approximately 10 minutes

Ingredients

- 3 cups sliced fresh strawberries
- ½ cup fresh basil, roughly chopped
- 2 Tbsp balsamic vinegar
- 1 Tbsp olive oil
- Pinch of salt and pepper

Method

1. Combine all ingredients in a bowl, taste, and adjust the vinegar, salt, and oil levels as required
2. Refrigerate until needed!

Nutritional information

- **Calories:** 76
- **Fat:** 3.8 grams
- **Protein:** 1.1 grams
- **Total carbs:** 10.4 grams
- **Net carbs:** 8 grams

Tagliatelle with garlic mushrooms

A simple pasta dish of silky tagliatelle, earthy mushrooms, garlic, and a dash of cream for a decadent weekend treat

Servings: 4

Time: approximately 30 minutes

Ingredients

- 15 oz dried tagliatelle
- 2 Tbsp olive oil
- 1 Tbsp butter
- 6 garlic cloves, finely chopped
- 4 cups sliced mushrooms, any variety (I like Swiss brown or Portobello)
- ⅓ cup dry white wine
- Salt and pepper
- Pinch of grated nutmeg
- 4 Tbsp cream

Method

1. Place a large saucepan of very salty water over a high heat, cover, and allow to boil
2. Add the tagliatelle to the boiling water and leave to cook as you prepare the mushrooms
3. Add the butter and olive oil to a sauté pan over a medium heat
4. Once the butter is melted and frothy, add the garlic and mushrooms and stir as they soften and the mushrooms reduce in size
5. Add the wine and allow to reduce for about 5 minutes
6. Add the salt, pepper, nutmeg, and cream, stir and remove from the heat
7. Drain the cooked pasta and reserve a cup of pasta water
8. Transfer the pasta to the pan with the mushrooms and add a dash of pasta water as you toss the pasta with tongs
9. Serve hot!

Nutritional information

- ***Calories:*** 552
- ***Fat:*** 16.3 grams
- ***Protein:*** 15.7 grams
- ***Total carbs:*** 82.4 grams
- ***Net carbs:*** 78.6 grams

Hearty Veggie, Bean and Barley Soup

This rustic soup features an abundance of veggies, white beans, barley, and rich broth. It's the perfect healthy Winter dinner, served with crusty bread

Servings: 6

Time: approximately 40 minutes

Ingredients

- 2 Tbsp olive oil
- 2 carrots, diced
- 2 onions, diced
- 3 celery sticks, diced
- 4 garlic cloves, roughly chopped
- 4 tomatoes, diced
- 2 zucchini, sliced
- 3 cups swiss chard, finely sliced
- 8 cups vegetable or chicken stock
- 1 cup pearl barley
- 2 cups cannellini beans
- Salt and pepper
- 1 bay leaf
- 1 rosemary sprig

Method

1. Add the olive oil to a stock pot over a medium heat
2. Add the carrots, onions, celery, garlic, tomatoes, zucchini, and swiss chard and stir to combine. Keep stirring for a few minutes as the veggies soften
3. Add the stock, barley, beans, salt, pepper, bay leaf, and rosemary, cover and leave to simmer for about 30 minutes or until the barley is tender
4. Serve steaming hot, with crusty bread

Nutritional information

- **Calories:** 348

- **_Fat:_** 10 grams
- **_Protein:_** 16.8 grams
- **_Total carbs:_** 56.4 grams
- **_Net carbs:_** 43 grams

Ratatouille

Ratatouille is a classic French dish with eggplants, tomatoes, zucchini, and herbs. Serve with crusty bread and a glass of red wine

Servings: 5

Time: approximately 1 hour and a half

Ingredients

- 2 Tbsp olive oil
- 1 onion, finely chopped
- 5 garlic cloves, finely chopped
- 2 bell peppers (red, yellow, or both), finely sliced
- 30 oz crushed canned tomatoes
- 2 large eggplants, thinly sliced
- 6 large tomatoes, thinly sliced
- 4 zucchinis, thinly sliced
- 2 Tbsp each fresh basil, thyme, and parsley, finely chopped
- Salt and pepper

Method

1. Preheat the oven to 400 degrees Fahrenheit
2. Drizzle the olive oil into a sauté pan over a medium-high heat
3. Add the onion, garlic, and bell peppers and stir as they soften for about 5 minutes
4. Add the crushed tomatoes, season with salt and pepper, stir to combine and leave to simmer for about 10 minutes
5. Remove the pan from the heat
6. Arrange the sliced eggplant, tomatoes, and zucchini in neat layers on top of the tomato sauce (they should be arranged in a repeated pattern)
7. Sprinkle the herbs and extra salt and pepper over the veggies
8. Cover the dish with foil and slip the pan into the oven to bake for about 40 minutes
9. Remove the foil and bake for a further 10-20 minutes or until the veggies are golden

Nutritional information

- ***Calories:*** 218
- ***Fat:*** 6 grams
- ***Protein:*** 6.3 grams
- ***Total carbs:*** 36.9 grams
- ***Net carbs:*** 24.8 grams

Roasted Bell Pepper Dip

Every Mediterranean feast needs a roasted bell pepper dip! This dip features bell peppers, onions, cashews and garlic

Servings: 5

Time: approximately 45 minutes

Ingredients

- 4 large red bell peppers, seeds removed
- 1 onion, finely sliced
- 4 garlic cloves, left unpeeled
- 3 Tbsp olive oil
- Salt and pepper
- ½ cup raw cashew nuts
- 1 tsp red wine vinegar

Method

1. Preheat the oven to 400 degrees Fahrenheit and line a baking tray with baking paper
2. Spread the bell peppers, onions, and garlic over the tray, rub with olive oil and sprinkle with salt and pepper
3. Slip the tray into the oven and roast the veggies for about 40 minutes or until very soft and almost charred
4. Transfer the peppers and onions into a food processor, and squeeze the soft garlic out of the skins into the food processor
5. Add the cashews and red wine vinegar and blend until very smooth

Serving suggestions: toasted pita bread, carrot sticks, or celery

Nutritional information

- **Calories:** 200
- **Fat:** 14.2 grams
- **Protein:** 4 grams
- **Total carbs:** 15.8 grams
- **Net carbs:** 11.8 grams

Conclusion

The Mediterranean diet is an intuitive way of eating, with a focus on fresh, seasonal, nutrient-dense foods. It's not about restricting certain food groups, but restricting processed food that doesn't offer nutritional value. You can enjoy wholesome bread, pasta, and grains as they provide excellent energy and fiber! No carb-cutting here! If you shop seasonally and get creative with vegetables, legumes, and grains, the possibilities are truly endless. I hope this book as given you some new favorite go-to recipes as well as the inspiration to create your own Mediterranean diet signature dishes! Your body and mind will thank you for making the transition to the Med diet. You'll enjoy clearer thinking, beautiful skin, a healthy heart, and will even drop any unwanted pounds! And hey…if you need a little more inspiration, you can always plan a holiday in the Mediterranean and learn from the locals!

Made in the USA
Monee, IL
25 February 2020